Contemporary Bioethics
Catholic Wisdom for a
Confused Culture

Contemporary Bioethics

Catholic Wisdom for a
Confused Culture

Edited by Marilyn E. Coors

℘

THE NATIONAL CATHOLIC BIOETHICS CENTER

Broomall, Pennsylvania

Published by
The National Catholic Bioethics Center
600 Reed Rd., Ste. 102
Broomall, PA 19008
Printed in the United States

Unless otherwise noted, scripture quotations are from Revised Standard Version of the Bible (RSV), © 1946, 1952, 1971, National Council of the Churches of Christ in the United States of America, and quotations from official Church documents are from the Vatican English translation, published online at www.vatican.va © Libreria Editrice Vaticana.

Library of Congress Control Number: 2024939890

ISBN 978-0-935372-81-6 (paperback)

Cover design by Nicholas Furton

Contents

EDITOR

Marilyn E. Coors, PhD, is an associate professor emerita of bioethics at the Center for Bioethics and Humanities at the University of Colorado Anschutz Medical Campus. She serves on the boards of directors for the National Catholic Bioethics Center and for Educating on the Nature and Dignity of Women (ENDOW).

CONTRIBUTORS

E. Christian Brugger, PhD, is a retired moral theologian living in Front Royal, Virginia.

Timothy Cardinal Dolan is the archbishop of New York.

Edward J. Furton, PhD, is the director of publications at the National Catholic Bioethics Center.

Elena Kraus, MD, PhD, practices maternal-fetal medicine at Mercy Clinic in St. Louis.

Joseph Meaney, PhD, is a senior fellow at the National Catholic Bioethics Center.

The Honorable Paul J. Ray is the director of the Thomas A. Roe Institute for Economic Policy Studies at the Heritage Foundation.

Christopher M. Reilly is a candidate for doctor of theology at Pontifex University and holds graduate degrees in theology, philosophy, and international and public affairs.

Rev. Columba Thomas, OP, MD, is a friar of the Province of St. Joseph and the McDonald Agape Fellow at the Edmund D. Pellegrino Center for Clinical Bioethics at Georgetown University.

Introduction

Marilyn E. Coors

Always being free to choose goodness is
demanding but it will make you into people with
a backbone who can face life, people with courage.
—Pope Francis

Jesus often taught deep truths using parables. His parable of the ten virgins illustrates the purpose of this book, which is to empower persons of faith to speak truthfully to contemporary bioethical issues in society. Ten virgins were invited to a wedding feast, and they each brought a lamp to watch for the arrival of the bridegroom. The five wise virgins were prepared with a flask of extra oil for their lamps, in case the bridegroom was delayed; the five foolish virgins were not. Upon the bridegroom's late arrival, the five "who were ready went in with him to the marriage feast; and the door was shut" (Matt. 25:10). The five whose oil was depleted went to buy more; when they returned, the doors to the feast were closed. They begged for admittance, but the bridegroom answered, "I do not know you" (Matt. 25:12). In this parable, those who were prepared followed this figure for Christ into the feast out of the messiness of culture. In case you are wondering why the wise virgins did not share their oil with the foolish ones, the oil of spiritual preparedness cannot be given to another.

It is my hope that this book will begin to fill the flasks for your lamps, so you can converse with friends and family, serve in churches and secular organizations, and vote from informed and reasoned positions grounded upon the light of truth.

Overview

In this anthology, nine interdisciplinary contributors address key bioethical topics that have implications for us, our countries, and potentially humankind. The topics were chosen through discussions with lay faithful to identify subjects about which they feel ill-equipped and would like to gain a deeper understanding. The teachings of Christ and the Church are the moral compass for this work. Where the Church has provided guidance on a topic, the authors include it in these chapters. Topics that are still under consideration by Church leaders and theologians are left open for further discussion. The audience for this book includes all readers who have an interest in the pressing issues presented here, whether they have a limited or an extensive background in bioethics.

Chapter 1 begins with an explanation of the importance of bioethics by Joseph Meaney. He describes the perfect storm of fast-paced biotechnological revolution and unprecedented cultural confusion. Meaney asserts that bioethics is the "conscience of technological civilization," which can be a remarkable force for good when based upon moral and intellectually sound principles.[1] Reverence for the unique dignity of the human person and respect for the created order of the world are the foci of the first chapter.

Timothy Cardinal Dolan follows in chapter 2 with an essay on human dignity, the foundation of morality and ethics. He affirms that every person possesses an inherent dignity, because he or she is created in the image and likeness of God. He tells a story of a young woman addicted to drugs and alcohol to illustrate that dignity does not depend on race, social status, passport, and so on, but on God's love for every one of his children.

I take a more scientific tack in chapter 3, as I simply define genome editing as specific point changes to DNA that treat disease or alter an organism. I develop the tale of the p53 gene, which is involved in human cancers, to illustrate the genetic and ethical complexity of altering humans. The concept of human dignity and the guiding principles of

---

1. Joseph Meaney, "The Importance of Bioethics," in *Contemporary Bioethics: Catholic Wisdom for a Confused Culture*, ed. Marilyn E. Coors (Broomall, PA: National Catholic Bioethics Center, 2024), 2.

the Popes, beginning with St. John Paul II in 1983 and continuing in the present with Francis, ground the evaluation of the ethical issues of safety, justice, and genetic enhancement.

E. Christian Brugger writes with wisdom in chapter 4 regarding sexual orientation, sexual behavior, and gender identity. He expresses sensitivity and mercy to individuals who experience gender confusion, and he emphasizes their personal dignity and need for compassionate care. Brugger provides the historical background for the intellectual and cultural dynamics leading to twenty-first-century cultural norms. He then exposes the errors in gender ideologies that deny the unity of body and soul, reject the complementarity of males and females, and refute the unitive and procreative nature of marriage.

While the notion of relativism is ubiquitous in our culture, many Christians are ill-equipped to recognize and respond to relativistic statements or beliefs. Edward Furton defines relativism in chapter 5 as the belief that persons can construct their own truths. He uses the disassociation of words and meanings, such as *existence, universe, marriage, good and evil*, and *tolerance*, to demonstrate relativism in culture. Furton asserts that if persons persist in redefining experience and creating their own reality, societal improvement will probably be beyond our grasp.

Elena Kraus, MD, explores the power of language to shape one's view of the world and change perceptions of morality in chapter 6. She describes the shift in the scientific definition of the beginning of life from fertilization to pregnancy, focused on the implantation of the early embryo, which was intended to rationalize abortion. Subsequently, Kraus explains how words influence the way physicians practice medicine and may contribute to health care disparities. She concludes with an account of the lack of civility in public discourse and encourages readers to call attention to irrationality or error in discussions and to present positive alternatives linked to the value of the human person at all stages.

In chapter 7, Christopher Reilly addresses the anxiety surrounding artificial intelligence and provides seven principles demonstrating how Christians can discern a path toward the best use of AI. Reilly warns that the constant use of technology can develop habits of manipulating persons or the environment for gain. He calls readers to faith and to the hope that free will and moral capacity will encourage applications of AI that contribute to true human development and overcome potential serious harms.

Paul Ray tells the story of St. Maximilian Kolbe's life as an example of Catholic social teaching (CST) in chapter 8. He portrays Kolbe as a man who lived as Christ and saw Christ in others. Ray explains what CST is and what it teaches—not politics or activism but an interior transformation of every person. The four principles of CST—dignity, subsidiarity, solidarity, and the common good—describe how we should live with love among other human beings. CST rejects atomistic individualism and calls people to work for their own good and the well-being of every other person.

Rev. Columba Thomas, OP, MD, closes the book with a discussion of vitalism and physician-assisted suicide, which are polar-opposite ethical choices in end-of-life care. Thomas gives an account of a patient, Joe, to illustrate the new hope and unprecedented complexity that medical care offers at the end of life. He goes on to define physician-assisted suicide, the legality of the practice, and the Church's teaching on this life-ending act. He concludes with a discussion of the intricacies of extraordinary and ordinary care to determine whether an intervention is obligatory or optional, according to Church teaching, in a person's circumstances. As a hospital chaplain, Thomas's stories about his patients are particularly effective in elucidating these difficult topics.

Going Forward

In Msgr. James Shea's book *From Christendom to Apostolic Mission*, he exhorts Christians to "understand our culture—its darkest depths as well as its most promising aspects—so that we can begin to know how to bring the light of Christ to it."[2] Shea explains that we are no longer living in a Judeo-Christian culture which provides society's basic assumptions of right and wrong, vice and virtue. Instead, we live in an apostolic age in which Christians typically embrace a spiritual and moral belief that is different from, and can be in opposition to, the culture in which we exist. This apostolic age will require us to prepare for opportunities to present a countercultural Christian vision in science, health care, politics, and everyday life. New depths of knowledge, grace, and courage will be required for every person to witness to the moral and ethical teachings of Christ and the Church in our world as it is.

---

2. James Shea, *From Christendom to Apostolic Mission: Pastoral Strategies for an Apostolic Age* (Bismarck, ND: University of Mary Press, 2020), 30.

1

The Importance of Bioethics

Joseph Meaney

Bioethics is arguably one of the most important practical and academic disciplines for the public and specialists to study today. This is a big claim, but it is easy to demonstrate. We are experiencing an unprecedented biomedical and scientific revolution that has been accelerating since the mid-twentieth century. For decades now, humanity has, for the first time, possessed immense raw scientific power, including the ability to destroy our world. The burning existential question is no longer the technical one, What can we achieve? Rather, there are ethical ones: What should be our medical and scientific goals? What limits need to be placed on research?

What Is Bioethics?

Ethics is the study of moral principles and actions. Bioethics applies ethics to living beings, especially when it comes to biomedical and technological interventions and research. It necessarily brings an interdisciplinary approach to ethics, since it involves medicine, science, and law as well as other areas, such as spiritual care.[1] Already in 1970, Van Rensselaer Potter underscored bioethics's broad scope when he defined it as "the science of

---

1.   Erica Laethem, "Why Bother with Bioethics?," in *Bioethics across the Life Span*, ed. Marilyn E. Coors (Philadelphia: National Catholic Bioethics Center, 2015), 5.

survival."[2] I especially like the concept of bioethics presented by Adriano Pessina. He refers to it as "the conscience of technological civilization."[3] Ethics is closely linked to the formation of conscience and the act of discerning what is right from what is wrong. The appropriate clinical and societal responses to medical problems should be implemented only after careful bioethical reflection, but in many cases, this does not happen, leading to such horrible violations of human rights as forcing patients to die alone without the bedside presence of loved ones or clergy, mistreating study participants, engaging in discriminatory prenatal genetic testing, directly hastening the deaths of vulnerable patients, and so on.

This problem of not seeing the need for science to be guided and governed by ethical bodies and sanctioned for ethical violations contributes to the many problems we face. Actions such as the National Institutes of Health's removal of mandatory review, by a special ethics advisory board, of extramural research grant and contract applications involving fetal tissue from elective abortions reinforce the caricature of bioethics as being mainly about doing a cursory review and writing permission slips for scientists or doctors to carry out their plans.[4] Unfortunately, many secular bioethicists and ethics committees do in fact often sign off, without any protest, on research or procedures that involve killing human embryos or other clearly unethical activities. In addition to being intrinsically wrong, these practices open a pandora's box of grave abuses against the dignity of the human person on a massive scale.

At the most personal level, however, bioethics is about medical decision-making for oneself or a loved one. Pope Pius XII acknowledged,

---

2. Van Rensselaer Potter, "Bioethics, the Science of Survival," *Perspectives in Biology and Medicine* 14.1 (Autumn 1970): 127–153, doi: 10.1353/pbm .1970.0015.

3. Adriano Pessina, *Bioetica: L'uomo sperimentale* (Milan: Bruno Mondatori, 1999), 22, quoted in Elio Sgreccia, *Personalist Bioethics: Foundations and Applications*, trans. John A. Di Camillo and Michael J. Miller (Philadelphia: National Catholic Bioethics Center, 2012), 23.

4. National Institute of Allergy and Infectious Diseases, "HHS Removes an Administrative Requirement for Human Fetal Tissue Research Proposals," National Institutes of Health, May 5, 2021, https://www.niaid.nih.gov /grants-contracts/hft-research-policy-change.

in a 1957 address to anesthesiologists, that the Church refuses to place stricter obligations on people than what is morally required, and that believers should have as much freedom as possible to act in conformity with the truth and what is morally good.[5] But it is not always easy to discern what is morally obligatory and what can be chosen or declined without any moral fault. To provide clear advice to patients or family members when they are distraught and vulnerable because of physical suffering or emotional distress, faithful Catholic bioethics has refined ethical principles such as double effect and the distinction between ordinary and extraordinary means. It is an exciting and a vital mission in our day, when so many scientific discoveries and cultural trends attack and exploit vulnerable human beings and the very order of nature.

Unfortunately, it can be very difficult to discern ordinary versus extraordinary means and what to choose or refuse among extraordinary means. That is one of the reasons the National Catholic Bioethics Center exists and provides a free ethical consultation service.[6] Thousands of clergy, religious, and laypeople have turned to the NCBC in these circumstances and experienced the benefits of having a trained ethicist assist them in their difficult discernment of what decisions to make.

The Source of Bioethics in the Order of Creation

Bioethics should be guided by a deep reverence for the unique dignity of the human person and a respect for the created order of the world. It is fundamental to sound bioethics that one has a true understanding of the human person, that is, an anthropology grounded in objective scientific observations and eternal truths. Most fundamentally, a key insight is the revealed understanding that human beings are created in the image and likeness of God, which endows every person with his or her incredible

---

5. Pius XII, "The Prolongation of Life: An Address to an International Congress of Anesthesiologists—November 24, 1957," trans. *The Pope Speaks* and *L'Osservatore Romano*, *National Catholic Bioethics Quarterly* 9.2 (Summer 2009): 325, doi: 10.5840/ncbq20099259.

6. To obtain free consultations by phone or email, visit National Catholic Bioethics Center, "Free Personal Consultation," accessed March 8, 2024, https://www.ncbcenter.org/ask-a-question.

dignity. It is also necessary to grasp that human beings are composite beings, combining mind, body, and soul.

Pope Francis has now issued two documents, *Laudato si'* and *Laudate Deum*, condemning a new technocratic paradigm that has led much of humanity to treat nature as an object of manipulation without respect for the order of creation. In these works, Francis explores the logical links between disrespecting our human ecology and abusing the natural ecology of the world: "The acceptance of our bodies as God's gift is vital for welcoming and accepting the entire world as a gift from the Father and our common home, whereas thinking that we enjoy absolute power over our own bodies turns, often subtly, into thinking that we enjoy absolute power over creation."[7]

Earlier, Pope Benedict XVI declared, in his encyclical *Caritas in veritate*, that the Catholic view of the intervention of science and technology on human beings and the natural world falls between two extremes: "When nature, including the human being, is viewed as the result of mere chance or evolutionary determinism, our sense of responsibility wanes. In nature, the believer recognizes the wonderful result of God's creative activity, which we may use responsibly to satisfy our legitimate needs, material or otherwise, while respecting the intrinsic balance of creation. If this vision is lost, we end up either considering nature an untouchable taboo or, on the contrary, abusing it. Neither attitude is consonant with the Christian vision of nature as the fruit of God's creation."[8]

I believe Benedict XVI was prophetic when he said that the great challenge of the future would be mankind's rejection of God the Creator. Today many scientists pursue experimental breakthroughs by sacrificing the lives of human embryos, completely heedless of the violation of the fundamental right to life of all human beings. Others radically alter the bodies of people surgically or hormonally without seeing that they are mutilating these poor persons and transgressing against human nature itself.

---

7. Francis, *Laudato si'* (May 25, 2015), n. 155. See also Francis, *Laudate Deum* (October 4, 2023).

8. Benedict XVI, *Caritas in veritate* (June 29, 2009), n. 48.

The Necessity of Catholic Bioethics

Our heterogeneous contemporary world is in dire need of morally and intellectually sound bioethics. We are in a kind of perfect storm, combining unprecedented cultural confusion about the nature and identity of the human person and a biotechnological revolution that is fast transforming science fiction into scientific possibility. The Catholic moral and intellectual tradition provides a treasure of insights that can help us make good decisions and offer strong arguments for better ethical guidelines in medical practice and scientific research. For all people, "the work of bioethics can and should be a service of charity, an act of love, where the authentic good of others is the goal. The purpose of bioethics is to help us be the kind of people we were made to be: people called to love."[9] Good bioethicists are guardians of what is sacred and inviolable in our brothers and sisters.

There has never been a time in human history when advancements in the biological sciences and technology have made radical interventions on the human body and the created world easier to carry out. These developments are a deep source of preoccupation for the Church. The *Doctrinal Note on the Moral Limits to Technological Manipulation of the Human Body* by the Doctrine Committee of the United States Conference of Catholic Bishops rightly observes that many biomedical breakthroughs—chemical, surgical, genetic, and so on—have made curing previously untreatable conditions and illnesses possible. This is very positive, but these discoveries can go against the fundamental "order in human nature we are called to respect"—for example, when the surgical and hormonal transformations of a person's body eliminate the characteristics of one sex and create the appearance of the opposite sex, or when healthy bodies are manipulated in a transhumanist quest for an eternal physical life or a new type of human being. To the contrary, "human nature deserves utmost respect since humanity occupies a singular place in the created order, being created in the image of God (Gen. 1:27)."[10]

---

9. Laethem, "Why Bother with Bioethics?," 21.
10. US Conference of Catholic Bishops Committee on Doctrine, *Doctrinal Note on the Moral Limits to Technological Manipulation of the Human Body* (March 20, 2023), 2; see also 10–11.

Secular bioethics tends to take the radical approach that the autonomous wishes of the patient simply should be accepted rather than ethically evaluated.[11] First, it is false to think we have anything approaching full autonomy, even as healthy adults. Human beings never cease to depend on others to help and guide them. More importantly, exercising one's autonomy counter to human dignity leads to death and the violation of other people's legitimate freedoms. There is definitely a balance to be respected. Forcing others to do what is right can be ethically corrosive and self-defeating, as it introduces evils in the fight against sin. On the other hand, complete permissiveness simply abandons people to fall easily into temptation and forsakes the weak and the vulnerable to be abused.

Ethical limits must go beyond just preventing injustice against others. We do need protections against making bad choices for ourselves while not destroying personal autonomy. Catholic wisdom takes autonomy, or free choice, very seriously and addresses what should be done to assist it. The Church places a great emphasis on how our conscience must be informed and guided. Our moral conscience needs to be educated from early childhood and throughout our lives.[12] Fallen human nature is an easily verifiable Christian doctrine, because we see, time and again, in ourselves and others, a tendency to choose evil, even though this is irrational and destructive.

---

11. See Tom L. Beauchamp and James F. Childress, *Principles of Biomedical Ethics*, 8th ed. (Oxford: Oxford University Press, 2019). In the United States, a very influential school of bioethics has been principlism. Beauchamp and Childress have advocated that four principles be applied to analyze all bioethical dilemmas: beneficence, nonmaleficence, respect for autonomy, and justice. Known as the Georgetown Principles, or more pejoratively as the Georgetown Mantra, an important criticism from a Catholic perspective is that the four principles do not put an adequate emphasis on the acting person. Ethicists can reach conclusions for or against certain actions that respect autonomy, for instance, but violate other important objective ethical norms.

12. *Catechism of the Catholic Church*, 2nd ed. (Washington, DC: US Conference of Catholic Bishops / Libreria Editrice Vaticana, 2018 update), nn. 1783–1784. All subsequent citations appear in the text.

Authentic civilization is rooted in morality and objective values. In fact, the dominant bioethical paradigm of societies is a key indicator of whether they are truly civilized. Scientific knowledge and development can be at the service of humanity or of barbarism, depending on the ethics that guides their application. The Nazi and Marxist revolutions are so morbidly fascinating because entire technologically advanced countries were enslaved to evil ideologies. They directly manifested what Pope St. John Paul II called a "culture of death," which is the opposite of true civilization.[13] One of the first things the Bolsheviks put in place after they seized power in Russia was legal abortion on demand. Even before he established the extermination camps, Hitler sterilized those he considered undesirable and euthanized the sick, especially those with inheritable genetic conditions.

The solutions to bioethical problems offered by the culture of death follow a pattern. They are technical interventions that provide a quick fix. Crisis pregnancy is solved by abortion. Pain and despair at the end of life are resolved by lethal injection or suicide. The brutal logic of the culture of death resolves problems by efficiently killing people. It brooks no restraints on selfish freedom and autonomy. A false understanding of compassion is one of the doorways to the abandonment of sound bioethics and true civilization. Too often, emotional responses to objectively terrible suffering make people believe they should commit injustices or ethical violations. By condoning abortion, euthanasia, or assisted suicide, we do not truly help struggling persons find a solution to their misery. Direct killing crosses a bright ethical line that goes beyond the justified and morally good relief of pain. Once accepted in the more extreme cases, the dreadful logic of abortion and euthanasia transforms healers into executioners.

The culture of life respects the preciousness of each person, and its solutions inevitably require much more time and energy. The pro-life support for a pregnant mother in crisis is tremendously more involved than a quick surgical procedure. When people are in pain or lonely and despairingly want to end their lives, the compassionate care they need is far more challenging and extensive than simply providing them with a

---

13. See John Paul II, *Evangelium vitae* (March 25, 1995), nn. 12, 21.

lethal injection or poison. Being pro-life means acknowledging that we are dependent on each other and have a duty to care for the vulnerable. Our Catholic vision of bioethics is that of a compassionate and objective search for what is true and good when ethical dilemmas arise in medicine or scientific research. A direct attack on the life of an innocent human being can never be sanctioned. Also, we cannot accept "the end justifies the means" reasoning that seeks to bring about a good end through evil acts. Time and again, such utilitarian thinking has led to terrible consequences, which are often referred to as the slippery slope.[14] In any case, it is terribly unethical to perform an evil act, even if one is motivated by good intentions.

Suffering is an evil, but it is not the supreme catastrophe that some make it out to be. It is also inevitable that we will face suffering in our lives. The Christian vision of redemptive suffering begins with the willingly accepted passion and death of Jesus Christ on the Cross to save us from our sins. The *Catechism of the Catholic Church* points to the belief that "Christ has given a new meaning to suffering: it can henceforth configure us to him and unite us with his redemptive Passion" (n. 1505). Suffering need not be meaningless, as many see or experience it. The saints teach us that it can be a strong means of growing in holiness if our hearts and wills respond with love and true compassion for others.

It is not easy to take up one's cross and follow the Lord, but this has been a key Christian insight for almost two millennia. Jesus loved to shake up our complacent lives and perspectives with paradoxes. The Beatitudes are full of apparently contradictory assertions, such as

---

14. A slippery slope describes the tendency to go further than initially intended once an action is initiated. Most people have fallen victim to the phenomenon. In many circumstances, fallen human nature resists limitations on certain activities. In bioethics there are many examples. One of the most tragic in several countries is the expansion of euthanasia and physician-assisted suicide. The first laws legally authorizing these practices generally have multiple stringent safeguards. Over time, more and more people are euthanized or kill themselves in violation of these safeguards. Rather than punishing those who break the law, however, the safeguards are often redefined as barriers to access and explicitly removed in subsequent legislation.

"blessed are those who mourn, for they shall be comforted" (Matt. 5:4). If Christ had not said that joyfully enduring insults and persecution for his sake would lead to great rewards in heaven, we might be more tempted to compromise with (or not be signs of contradiction to) the powerful ideologies of our age.

All this brings us back to civilization and bioethics. To be uncivilized is about something much deeper than rudeness or a lack of refinement. A failed civilization does not pass the test of treating the most weak and vulnerable ethically. Justice and objective values are pillars of civilization. Abandoning either, one falls into the arbitrariness that is a hallmark of barbarism. There can be a civilization of love but not one of ethical relativism. Technological advancement and biomedical practice must be guided by civilized bioethics. If they are not, then terrible human rights abuses inevitably will follow.

Bioethics can be a remarkable force for good and the Gospel of life. When it is perverted, however, it loses the vital connection that promotes the unique dignity of the human person in a compassionate and truthful way. Some scientists and doctors are tempted to play God and disregard our just limitations as created beings. Good bioethicists are guardians of what is sacred and inviolable in our brothers and sisters. They are defenders of the dignity of the human person and our created world.

2

What Does It Mean to Be Human?

Timothy Cardinal Dolan

A Doctrine with Real Consequences

In July 2002, I led a group of about three hundred young people from the Archdiocese of St. Louis to Toronto for World Youth Day, an idea which came from the genius of Pope St. John Paul II, who, every two or three years, would invite young people from all over the planet to join him for five days of prayer, catechesis, faith sharing, and friendship at different locations across the globe.

It was my happy task, in the midst of a million young folks, to offer a catechesis on three different days to about three hundred people from Canada, Ireland, England, Australia, India, and the United States at a parish setting in the suburbs of Toronto. On the third day, at the close of our final catechesis, I asked my group if anyone wanted to speak publicly about if or how this World Youth Day had transformed his or her life. After a pause of a few seconds, a young woman in the back corner stood up and approached one of the two available microphones.

"Yes! This event has not only changed my life. It has *saved* my life!" she began. "See, I was living on the streets of Detroit, under a highway overpass. I ran away from home seven years ago, when I was thirteen. I'm

---

A previous version of this chapter was published as "The Dignity of a Human Person: A Catholic Doctrine," *Church Life Journal*, April 4, 2016, https://church lifejournal.nd.edu/articles/the-dignity-of-a-human-person-a-catholic-doctrine/. Reprinted with permission.

addicted to alcohol and heroin"—with that she showed her bare arms, so we could see the bruises and scabs from the needles—"and have been a prostitute for years to support those habits. Been in jail on and off for shoplifting. Anyway, the youth group at my parish kind of adopted me. Took me in, got me some counseling and treatment, even a room, and invited me to this World Youth Day. I came on a dare, nothing better to do, figuring I'd come up here, break from the group, stay in Canada, and go back to my old way of life. But something happened here. I've met an old man who tells me he loves me. Oh, I'm used to men telling me they love me as they give me $50. But this old man seems to mean it. This old man tells me God also loves me. This old man tells me I'm the apple of God's eye, his work of art, made in his image, redeemed by his Son; that I'm so special that God wants me on his lap for all eternity.

"This old man has given me a reason to live," she said, wrapping up. "My life has not just been changed, but *saved*."

Of course, the old man was John Paul II, who, although already stooped and shaky, unable to walk, quivering and drooling, was there at World Youth Day and had spoken such words to the millions of young people. That twenty-year-old addict-prostitute had just confessed her belief in the *Catholic doctrine of the dignity of the human person*. This doctrine obviously had real consequences: her failing to understand how it applied to her life nearly ended her life. But once she understood it, not only was her life saved, but it began to flourish.

Today, I fear, much of secularized Western culture is as lost as this young woman was before her encounter with John Paul II. Our culture has not passed on the foundation of human dignity and equality, both of which are based on theological ideas. As the *Catechism of the Catholic Church* teaches, man "alone is called to share, by knowledge and love, in God's own life. ... This is the fundamental reason for his dignity. ... Being in the image of God the human individual possesses the dignity of a person, who is not just something, but someone."[1]

God made me in his own image and likeness; I am worth the Precious Blood of his only begotten Son; I am God's work of art; He calls

---

1. *Catechism of the Catholic Church*, 2nd ed. (Washington, DC: US Conference of Catholic Bishops / Libreria Editrice Vaticana, 2018 update), nn. 356–357.

me by name; He knows me better than I know myself; He loves me so powerfully, personally, and passionately that He wants me to spend eternity with him; I have come from him and am destined to return to him forever. As St. Irenaeus chanted, "The glory of God is a living man."[2] The human person is of such worth that God himself took on our nature at the *Incarnation*; the human person has such dignity that God's Son died lest he or she perish in what we call the *redemption*.

As I used to comment to those assembled for the sacrament of Confirmation, if we really believed what the Church teaches on the dignity of the human person, think of what a difference it would make in the way we treat ourselves, in the way we treat others. It would be *lifesaving*. Ask my friend in Toronto. Also ask our culture, one so obviously in desperate need of better answers to the question of this chapter.

Allow me to make five observations about this.

The Church's Defense of the Doctrine

The first observation is about the Church's defense of the doctrine of the dignity of the human person at the core of what we call the Judeo-Christian tradition. True enough, the dignity of creature and creation itself was gravely ruptured in this normative narrative, but as we recall on the feast of the Immaculate Conception, even then God already had in mind a grand restoration of the pinnacle of his creation, the human person.

It is so tenderly evident in the Law and the prophets, in the teaching of Jesus and St. Paul. It has given rise to Christian morality, which startled the brutality of the Roman world with its emphasis on the protection of life, respect for the person, care for the vulnerable, and defense of women, babies, children, family, elders, and even slaves. It gave rise to the greatest system of health care, education, and charity the world has ever known, giving us great saints and other holy men and women whose solicitude for the little ones, the oppressed, and the struggling captures our imagination to this day. It inspired a Bartolomé de las Casas, a Martin Luther King Jr., a Dorothy Day as they recognized the human person as a reflection

---

2. Irenaeus, *Against Heresies*, trans. Alexander Roberts and William Rambaut, in *Ante-Nicene Fathers*, vol. 1, ed. Alexander Roberts et al. (Christian Literature, 1885; New Advent, n.d.), IV.20.7.

of the divine, and it led them to the radical claim that even those to whom the culture had denied fundamental human equality—such as the slave, native American, or person of a racial minority—were created in the image and likeness of God in precisely the same way as any other human being was.

The caricature of the Church is that it had to be dragged kicking and screaming into the noble enterprise of defending human rights. More sober voices now conclude that the forces of the Enlightenment and of the French Revolution, untethered from this Catholic doctrine of the dignity of the human person, are partly the cause of horrors such as the gulags, camps, and killing fields of the last century, and that they are at the center of our own century's horrors. Figures like la Cases, King, and Day reveal a human rights tradition that has its foundations in, again, *theological* claims.

And this fact is not lost on everyone. A few years ago, I received one of the more surprising invitations I ever have: to come to England for the eight hundredth anniversary of the *Magna Carta*.

"Why an American? And why me, a Catholic Archbishop?" I asked the organizer.

"Because the United States is an inheritor of the tradition begun by the *Magna Carta*," he replied. "And because the *Magna Carta* was composed by an archbishop, and because it flows from the teaching of the Church on human rights and justice."

It is now clear that the Catholic Church is the world's most dramatic defender of the dignity of the person and radical human equality. Such should hardly startle one versed in the Catholic doctrine of the dignity of the human person.

A Positive Vision of the Good

Too often the Church's defense of what it means to be human is understood as a no to something. And while there are indeed times it is very important to explicitly reject attacks on fundamental human equality, our faith teaches us that our heavenly Father looks upon us, sees his Son, and smiles. Every human life beams with the transcendent and hints at the beyond, at a faith that affirms everything that is decent, noble, and uplifting in the human drama.

And here is my second point: the Catholic doctrine of the dignity of the human person prompts a resounding yes to whatever affirms the truth, beauty, and goodness inherent in us and in our world. This is the Christian humanism of giants such as Eramus and St. Thomas More. So too the history of the Church has produced the poetry of Dante and the art of Caravaggio, the sculpture of Michelangelo and the music of Mozart, the research of Mendel and the discoveries of Columbus, the charm of St. Francis and frescoes of Giotto.

The Church is into affirming not denouncing, raising up not putting down, encouraging not condemning. As Bishop Robert Barron claims in his marvelous and exciting *Catholicism* series, the Church is all about a yes to all that is true, beautiful, and good in the human project. The Church says no only to something or someone that would negate the true, the beautiful, or the good in the human person. And a no to another no results in a yes!

A Doctrine Which Calls Us to Act

Third, not least because this positive vision of the doctrine has real consequences (saving lives when present and driving people to despair when it is not), we have a moral imperative to *act*. If it is true that we are temples of the Holy Spirit—that we are vessels of the divine and icons of the Trinity, that, when God the Father looks at us, He sees the face of his Son, Jesus—*actions* must follow from this. We ought to behave as if we really think it is true.

As Pope Benedict XVI remarked during his apostolic visit to his homeland, this is the transition from the *is* to the *ought* upon which our moral decisions and actions are grounded.[3] If we are divinized, reflections of God created in his image and likeness—there is the *is*—then we *ought* to treat ourselves and others only with respect, love, honor, and care.

- If the preborn baby in the womb, from the earliest moments of his or her conception, *is* a human person—an *is* that comes not from the *Catechism* but from the biology textbook used

---

3. Benedict XVI, "The Listening Heart: Reflections on the Foundations of Law" (Reichstag Building, Berlin, September 22, 2011).

by any sophomore in high school—then that baby's life *ought* to be cherished and protected.

- If an immigrant or refugee *is* a child of God, worth the price of the life of God's only begotten Son, then we *ought* to render him or her honor and a welcome, not a roar of hate, clenched fists, and gritted teeth in response to the latest campaign slogan from a candidate appealing to the nativistic side of our nature.

- If a young woman suffering from gender dysphoria *is* a human being—created with a body-soul dyad that reflects the image and likeness of her Creator—then we *ought* to do all we can to help her understand the goodness of her created body, and we *ought* to work within the Church's broad tradition to help her understand the myriad ways one can express what it means to be a woman.

- If even a man on death row has a soul, is a human person—an *is* that cannot be erased even by beastly crimes he may have committed—then we *ought* not to strap him to a gurney and inject him with poison until he is dead and tell ourselves that this counts as a kind of justice.

- If a human being is sick, frail, and suffering from cognitive injury or decline—she *is* a vulnerable member of the human family who bears the face of Christ as the least among us—and then we *ought* to show her genuine and nonviolent compassion ("suffer with" her), care, and hospitality.

It is not without irony that, as I look back at my time in Canada as such a great victory for human dignity and equality, at the moment I put this essay together, our neighbors to the north are offering assisted suicide to everyone from veterans suffering from post-traumatic stress disorder to the poor who cannot afford proper housing to those who need to wait too long for needed medical procedures. How desperately we need the Catholic doctrine of the dignity of the human person! And how desperately we need to move from the *is* to the *ought*! The very lives of the most vulnerable members of the human family are at stake.

We Are Given Our Identity

A fourth observation: in an age of obsession about self-created identity (and, not accidentally, one dominated by massive amounts of anxiety and depression) the Catholic doctrine of the dignity of the human person insists that our identity *is a given*: we *are* children of God, his creation, modeled in his own image, destined for eternity. That is our *identity*.

We are *not* identified with our urges, our flaws, our status, our possessions, or our utility. John Paul II taught that the great heresy today is that we stress *having* and *doing* over *being*.[4] My identity, my personhood, my *is-ness* and the respect such an *is-ness ought* to engender do *not* depend on whether I have a green card, a stock portfolio, a job, a home, or even a college diploma. Nor does my identity depend upon to whom I am sexually attracted or upon race, religion, gender, or health insurance, but upon my essence as a child of God.

So, to the recovering alcoholic crying in the confessional at St. Patrick's Cathedral after a two-day binge back in Manhattan, "I am a hopeless drunk," we reply, "No, you are a child of God, made in his likeness, loved passionately and personally by a God who claims you as his own, but who happens to have an addiction to alcohol." So, to the protestors outside St. Patrick's who, disagreeing with the Church's defense of traditional marriage, yell at me, "I am gay, why do you hate me?" I respond, "Nice to meet you. As a matter of fact, I love you; you *are* God's work of art, the apple of his eye, embraced by a God who passionately loves you, who happens to have a same-sex attraction." Who we *are* is of infinitely more significance than what we have, do, or drink or to whom we are sexually attracted.

As he was wont to do, Benedict XVI gave a fresh twist to this approach to morality. Again in his address before the German parliament, the Holy Father spoke about the need to reverence both the external environment of *creation* and the internal ecology of the *Creator*. Thank God, the Pontiff remarked, we creatures have learned, albeit the hard way, that

---

4.   John Paul II, *Sollicitudo rei socialis* (December 30, 1987), n. 28.

the environment of our earth has a built-in balance, a fragile structure and equilibrium. Creation has an order about it, a delicate stasis that should never be tampered with or polluted. The "Green Pope"—as Benedict XVI has been called—went on to remind us as well that, just as there is an integrity in *creation* that must be safeguarded, and a law of nature that is evident to us who are tempted to abuse it, so is there an order, a balance, a coherence innate in *creatures*, in the human person, that is protected by a *natural* law which must be heeded.

Listen to his words: "The importance of ecology is no longer disputed. We must listen to the language of nature and we must answer accordingly. Yet I would like to underline a point that seems to me to be neglected. … There is also an ecology of man. Man too has a nature that he must respect and that he cannot manipulate at will. Man is not merely self-creating freedom. Man does not create himself. … His will is rightly ordered if he respects his nature, listens to it and accepts himself for who he is."[5]

Resisting a Slide into Heresy

Here is my final observation, number five, again on this moral journey from the *is* to the *ought*: we have been talking about a doctrine, the dignity of the human person. The right teaching of any doctrine is called *orthodoxy*; the wrong understanding of any doctrine is called *heresy*. Hilaire Belloc reminds us that a heresy usually is not a denial of a doctrine but an obsessive exaggeration of one element of it.[6] So can our orthodox expression, promotion, and defense of this Catholic doctrine of the dignity of the human person become heretical if we wrongheadedly exaggerate only one of its carefully balanced parts.

The orthodox insistence upon the dignity of the human person, with the logical corollary that every person deserves dignity and respect, becomes as a matter of fact heretical if it sinks into a narcissistic demand for whatever pleasure or right to which I feel I am entitled. For the same doctrine that gives rise to a grand tradition of respect for human rights also gives us the call to *duty* and *responsibility*. As John Paul II often

---

5. Benedict XVI, "Listening Heart."
6. Hilaire Belloc, *The Great Heresies* (San Francisco: Ignatius Press, 2017), 71.

preached, "Freedom consists not in doing what we like, but in having the right to do what we ought."[7]

It can also become heretical if only certain aspects of the doctrine are emphasized with the goal of advancing a particular secular political narrative or agenda. The Catholic doctrine of the dignity of the human person transcends secular politics, urging members of all parties and interest groups to move from the *is* to the *ought* not because of idolatrous political agendas but because they recognize and support the fundamental dignity and equality of all human beings wherever we find them.

Conclusion

I started with a young woman in Toronto. Let me conclude with a young man back in St. Louis, my hometown. I grew up with Dan, let me call him, and he was a boyhood buddy whom I lost track of during college and seminary. I had heard Dan had gone to Vietnam and come back with a scrambled brain; he was into drugs, living on the street. I often thought of Dan and wondered how he was. A couple weeks after my ordination, Dan shows up at the rectory of my first parish, clean, well-dressed, smiling, with a young woman he introduced to me as his fiancée. During our chat, he brought up his grimy past.

"Tim, you may have heard that I've been messed up big time. I was literally in the gutter, drinking, popping, smoking, injecting whatever I could. I had hit bottom. Late one night, in a warehouse down off Biddle Street, on the riverfront, another druggie and I had landed a stash of cheap heroin. We were ready to needle it in when the other guy says, 'Dan, I dare you. You and I are both trash. We're both done with life. We have no tomorrow. Let's go out on a high. I dare you! I'll give you ten seconds to come up with a decent reason why we're here, or, I dare you, let's give each other a triple dose of this stuff and call it quits.'

"Tim, what could I do?" Dan went on. "I had ten seconds to give him—and me—a reason to keep going. In desperation, all that came to my blurry mind was the third question in the *Baltimore Catechism* that you and I learned in second grade at Holy Infant grade school way back.

---

7. John Paul II, homily (Oriole Park at Camden Yards, Baltimore, October 8, 1995), n. 7.

I blurted it out: 'Why did God make you? God made me to know Him, love Him, and serve Him in this life, and to be happy with Him forever in the next.' The other guy held the needle suspended and looked at me. 'Say that again.' I did. He thought a minute, and finally answered, 'Not bad. I'll take it.' And I'm still here!"

That is the doctrine of the dignity of the human person. It saved Dan's life; it saved the life of our young friend in Toronto. The Church's vision is nothing less than lifesaving.

It is up to us not only to defend it in the public sphere but to build the kinds of ecclesial and theological communities that give people from Toronto to St. Louis (and, indeed, to all nations) a shot at understanding and internalizing it. This means not just understanding that the dignity of the human person is a theological doctrine but intentionally building communities around this theological doctrine, communities which form people who really believe it is true—both about themselves and about every single human being.

3

Modifying Life:
Genome Editing for Better or Worse

Marilyn E. Coors

*Technological development has also brought about an attack,
often unwittingly, on human nature itself. Long-standing
assumptions about what it means to be human are under
siege. ... There needs to be a re-articulation of the truth that can
provide those who are languishing under the malnourishment
of the modern spiritual diet a way out of their predicament.*

—Msgr. James Shea

In this technological culture, many people seek understanding and moral
clarity regarding new innovations. Genome editing is a striking example
of such a new technology, and Church teachings provide important guidance. Genome editing is a simple way to make precise changes in DNA
sequences and carry out genetic research cheaply. It is also incredibly
powerful. This formidable technology's combination of attributes (easy,
cheap, and powerful) warrants a deeper moral and ethical analysis. In
2003, scientists completed the Human Genome Project, which decoded
the human genome (all DNA in an organism) and generated the capacity
to read DNA; now genome editing provides the tools to rewrite the DNA
sequences of plants, animals, and humans. The technological capacity to
rewrite the code of life resembles the aspiration of Adam and Eve to possess all knowledge: "For God knows that when you eat of it, your eyes will

be opened, and you will be like God, knowing good and evil" (Gen. 3:5). While God created man and woman to be cocreators and stewards with him (Gen. 1:28, 2:19–20), Adam and Eve chose to become creators on their own. In many ways, the new innovations in science and technology present humankind with a similar choice.

Jennifer Doudna, who, along with Emmanuelle Charpentier, won the Nobel Prize in Chemistry in 2020 for developing genome editing, recognized the potential for good and evil in this new technology almost immediately. She reported a timely nightmare during which she walked into a room and saw a person who said to her, "I want to understand your new technology."[1] The person looked up, and Doudna knew it was Adolf Hitler. At that moment, she starkly realized that genome editing in the wrong hands could cause great harm rather than the intended benefit, which is to develop cures and treatments for genetic disease. She subsequently gathered scientists from around the world to discuss limiting genetic alterations that would be inheritable or difficult to control. Given the ethical concerns she expressed, Pope Francis appointed Doudna and Charpentier to the Pontifical Academy of Sciences in 2021. Francis encouraged dialogue with scientific experts and cautioned geneticists to pursue scientific advancement only through means that do not contribute to the throwaway culture or exploit human beings as objects for use.[2]

Science of Genome Editing

To conduct a sound ethical analysis, it is necessary to understand the science of genome editing. The current group of technologies included under the category of genome editing are CRISPR-Cas9 as well as base and prime editing, and there certainly will be more innovations in the future. With this technology, it is possible to reshape medical treatments, develop treatments or cures for genetic disorders like HIV, Huntington's

---

1. Terry Gross, "CRISPR Scientist's Biography Explores Ethics of Rewriting the Code of Life," *Fresh Air*, March 8, 2021, https://www.npr.org /sections/health-shots/2021/03/08/974751834/crispr-scientists-biography -explores-ethics-of-rewriting-the-code-of-life.
2. Francis, Address to the participants in the meeting "Faith and Science: Toward COP26" (October 4, 2021).

disease, sickle cell anemia, beta thalassemia, cystic fibrosis, and cancer,[3] edit animal organs for transplantation, study gene function, create gene drives to control insect vectors of diseases and agricultural pests,[4] and genetically modify livestock and crops.[5] Along with these promising applications, there are concerns regarding scientific risks, societal implications, moral issues, and challenges to what it means to be human.[6]

Many Catholics and people of other religions feel that our churches avoid discussing the ethical issues surrounding genome editing. Bioethics can be confusing for many people of faith. Some of this stems from a lack or inconsistency of knowledge among priests and pastors, which can undermine trust. As a result, there is a void of information and understanding on the part of the faithful regarding the Church's position on genome editing. Pope St. John Paul II gave an address discussing the morality of genetic technology to the World Medical Association in 1983, which established the guiding principles for evaluating the ethics of genetic modification interventions. The ethical reflection and guidance contained in that address are reflected in the later writings of Pope Benedict XVI and Francis and in the instruction *Dignitas personae*. John Paul II states, "A strictly therapeutic intervention whose explicit objective is the healing of various maladies such as those stemming from deficiencies of chromosomes will, in principle, be considered desirable, provided it is directed to the true promotion of the personal well-being of man and does not infringe on his integrity or worsen his conditions of life."[7] He goes on to discuss respect for life, marginalization, and enhancement. We

---

3. Jennifer A. Doudna, "The Promise and Challenge of Therapeutic Genome Editing," *Nature* 578.7794 (February 2020): 229–236, doi: 10.1038/s41586-020-1978-5.

4. George J. Annas et al., "A Code of Ethics for Gene Drive Research," *CRISPR Journal* 4.1 (February 2021): 19–24, doi: 10.1089/crispr.2020.0096.

5. Nicholas Kalaitzandonakes et al., "The Economics and Policy of Genome Editing in Crop Improvement," *Plant Genome* 16.2 (June 2023), e20248, doi: 10.1002/tpg2.20248.

6. Congregation for the Doctrine of the Faith (CDF), *Dignitas personae* (September 8, 2008), nn. 1–37.

7. John Paul II, Address at the Conclusion of the Thirty-Fifth General Assembly of the World Medical Association (November 17, 1983), n. 6.

will return to this document and others as we discuss three ethical issues and the moral challenges of genome editing.

Applications of Human Genome Editing

Genome editing can make specific point changes to DNA via enzymes in non-dividing body cells (somatic cells) such as tissues or organs. The hope is to treat or cure disease. It can convert a disease-causing segment of DNA (one base pair) into a functioning one, enabling the targeted body cells to operate properly. Alterations to a patient's own cells can occur inside the body (in vivo) or outside of the body (in vitro) and then be returned to the patient. These therapeutic changes occur in an individual patient for potential benefit and cease to exist at a person's death. In 1998 John Paul II expressed a positive vision of genetic medicine in an address to the Pontifical Academy for Life: "I therefore hope that the conquest of this new continent of knowledge, the human genome, will mean the discovery of new possibilities for victory over disease and will never encourage a selective attitude towards human beings."[8]

Genome editing can also alter the DNA of reproductive cells, for example, eggs or sperm (gametes) or human embryos (via in vitro fertilization and prenatal genetic diagnosis), in an attempt to treat genetic disease or enhance normal function. Changes to reproductive cells are permanent and do not cease to exist when the patient dies. These changes are passed down to future generations and become part of the human gene pool. Human embryo manipulation is illicit according to Catholic teaching, because "it invariably causes the death of embryos and is consequently gravely illicit: 'research, in such cases, irrespective of efficacious therapeutic results, is not truly at the service of humanity.'"[9] In accord with this, Francis emphatically stated at a Vatican-organized conference highlighting global awareness of Huntington's disease, "Some branches of research use human embryos, inevitably causing their destruction, but we know

---

8.   John Paul II, "Introduction," in *Human Genome, Human Person and the Society of the Future: Proceedings of the Fourth Assembly of the Pontifical Academy for Life*, ed. Juan de Dios Vial Correa and Elio Sgreccia (Vatican City: Libreria Editrice Vaticana, 1999), 9.

9.   CDF, *Dignitas personae*, n. 32.

that no ends, even noble in themselves—such as a predicted utility for science, for other human beings or for society—can justify the destruction of human embryos."[10] Scientifically, the safety risks of altering embryos before implantation are significant if not insurmountable because of the possibility of unintended consequences (accidental off-target alterations) and the unknown interrelationships of all genes and genetic diseases.[11]

Being Human

The potential of genome editing to alter ourselves and other species calls into question what it means to be human. Accordingly, we look to the primacy of human dignity as the fundamental value to guide genomic medicine and research. The Catholic notion of human dignity entails three basic concepts: "(1) respect for life, (2) the integral union of bodily and spiritual elements in human the person, (3) human liberty."[12] The first, respect for life, prohibits research on human embryos and zygotes, as discussed above. Respect for life also disallows any intervention that reduces human life to an object, rather than recognizing each person's inestimable value, intelligence, and liberty as "created in the image and likeness of God" (Gen. 1:26). By *object* is meant the instrumental treatment of the human person or embryo as a tool of research for utilitarian purposes. This includes research for which there are no limits concerning what experimental manipulations scientists can perform.

A second aspect of human dignity is integral unity. The Catholic Church teaches that the human person, created in the image of God, embraces body and soul united as one integral person. Given the fantasies of social media and the false promises of an alternative reality where

---

10. Felix N. Codilla, "Pope Francis Cautions against Dangers of Genetic Manipulation That Can Create 'Throwaway Culture,'" *Christian Post*, May 23, 2017, https://www.christianpost.com/news/pope-francis-cautions-against-dangers-of-genetic-manipulation-that-can-create-super-humans.html.

11. Jeffrey R. Botkin, "The Case for Banning Heritable Genome Editing," *Genetics in Medicine* 22.3 (November 2019): 487–489, doi.: 10.1038/s41436-019-0696-6.

12. Joseph Zycinski, "Bioethics, Technology and Human Dignity: The Roman Catholic Viewpoint," *Acta Neurochirurgica* 98 suppl (2006): 3.

the mind exists but the body is ignored or devalued, this teaching takes on additional importance in assessing genetic alterations. Applications of genome editing are moral when the outcome entails benefit for the entire person, not enhancing mind over body or the reverse. Thus, this teaching excludes the creation of new forms of humans, for example, persons with enhanced cognitive skills or strength to dominate aspects of society or with diminished intellect to perform undesirable or dangerous tasks for society (not possible at the present state of science). The *Catechism of the Catholic Church* is clear: "For this reason, man may not despise his bodily life. Rather he is obliged to regard his body as good and to hold it in honor since God has created it and will raise it up on the last day."[13]

A third aspect of human dignity is liberty. St. Paul's letter to the Galatians provides us with a deep understanding of the essence of Christian liberty, which humans have as beings possessing intellect and free will in the image of God: "For freedom Christ has set us free; stand firm therefore, and do not submit again to the yoke of slavery" (Gal. 5:1). Modern-day slavery could entail pride, greed, fear, addiction, obsession with power and control, and so on. Paul goes on to explain what is meant by true freedom: "For you were called to freedom, brothers. Only do not use your freedom as an opportunity for the flesh, but through love, serve one another" (Gal. 5:13). In this letter, Paul also acknowledges that all lawful things are not always good for others and that freedom has a social dimension that involves the common good. Thus, the paradox of freedom is that it does not mean acting in our own self-interest to attain fame or fortune, but acting in service to others. Genuine freedom is the everyday pursuit to advance the common good, for example, the advancement of science to develop new treatments and cures. Francis explains that "freedom is very different from license; it is not found in giving into our own selfish desires, but instead leads us to serve others. 'True freedom is fully expressed in love.'"[14]

---

13. *Catechism of the Catholic Church*, 2nd ed. (Washington, DC: US Conference of Catholic Bishops/Liberia Editrice Vaticana, 2018 update), n. 364.
14. Christopher Wells, "The Pope at Audience: Freedom Is Born in God's Love, Grows in Charity," Vatican News, October 20, 2021, https://www.vaticannews.va/en/pope/news/2021-10/pope-francis-general-audience-paul-galatians-freedom-charity.html.

The recent declaration *Dignitas infinita* presents a thorough biblical and historical clarification of the aspects of human dignity with contemporary moral relevance. The declaration states that the concept of dignity can be misused to justify new rights which oppose the fundamental right to life, such as those discussed in this chapter and others: "This perspective identifies dignity with an isolated and individualistic freedom that claims to impose particular subjective desires and propensities as 'rights' to be guaranteed and funded by the community. However, human dignity cannot be based on merely individualistic standards, nor can it be identified with the psychophysical well-being of the individual. Rather, the defense of human dignity is based on the constitutive demands of human nature, which do not depend on individual arbitrariness or social recognition."[15] This elucidation of liberty is especially important as we consider the power of genome editing, which has the potential to fundamentally change the nature of human beings, our planet, and future generations.

Ethics Concerns

Safety

Determinations of safety entail the analysis of the risks, harms, and benefits of genome editing for human health and the environment. The alteration of a given gene could have a discreet intended effect that improves health or function for a person, plant, or organism. However, genes are interconnected, meaning that most genes seem to have multiple functions in addition to their known functions when activated in conjunction with other genes. At this stage of genetic science, scientists do not have complete knowledge regarding all associations among genes, which further complicates deciphering the genome. As a result, a genetic alteration could have unexpected or even deleterious effects on a patient which are difficult to predict or understand. Likewise, an alteration could have radically different outcomes for different individuals. An alteration that is safe for one person might not be safe for another, even in a well-studied gene, making safety difficult to assess.

---

15. Dicastery for the Doctrine of the Faith, *Dignitas infinita* (April 8, 2024), n. 25.

An illustrative example of this complexity is the story of the gene p53, which is involved in many human cancers.[16] P53 detects damage to DNA in cells and triggers the repair of the damage or, when DNA cannot be repaired, causes those cells to stop reproducing or die, helping to prevent cancer. By correlation, an increase in p53 activity should protect against cancer. In 2002 an unintended increase in the p53 gene in a laboratory experiment with mice produced a strain of mice which had normal development and a reduced incidence of tumors, compared with normal control mice. However, the altered mice aged more rapidly (osteoporosis, atrophy of muscle, and weight loss) and died sooner than the normal mice. This accidental research in a well-studied gene confirmed that p53 did indeed prevent cancer, but it also adversely affected aging, which was unknown at the time of the experiment. This research example confirmed that our genomes are not always easy to understand or completely safe to alter.

The above account of the complexity of the genome raises the issue of informed consent for procedures utilizing genome editing, which is rarely mentioned in the relevant literature. Informed consent is an ethical and legal requirement for persons undergoing a medical procedure or participating in research. It is a process of decision-making intended to protect the rights of the patient and shield him or her from undue harm. Informed consent entails a conversation between a medical professional and the potential patient to ensure the understanding of the relevant medical facts and risks involved, followed by the permission of the patient to undergo the procedure free of coercion or undue outside influence. Given the incomplete understanding of the genome and the potential for off-target mistakes, an accurate description of the risks involved is very difficult. While all medical procedures involve risk, the added unknowns surrounding genome editing create heightened obligations to ascertain understanding during the informed consent process.

Access and Justice

Human genome editing raises the ethical issue of equality of access. Costs and allocation play an important role in the United States and globally in

---

16. Judith Campisi, "Between Scylla and Charybdus: P53 Links Tumor Suppression and Aging," *Mechanisms of Ageing and Development* 123.6 (March 2002): 567–573, doi: 10.1016/s0047-6374(02)00006-4.

health care access. Access to health care includes both the opportunity for insurance coverage and the prospect of obtaining a needed genomic therapy. Any new and expensive therapy may be accessible only to wealthy individuals and developed countries, probably increasing existing health disparities among groups and nationalities. For example, if persons cannot pay for treatment that is available, access is denied. Or if a treatment is covered by insurance but not available in a region or country for logistical reasons (lack of clinics, refrigeration, or technology), there is no fair access. Of course, during research trials or clinical development of a new therapy, there is often a lag in coverage, access, or affordability. This is tragic but can qualify as just if remedies, over time, are found for the issue of lack of access.

Research is another area that sometimes reflects inequality among ethnicities or groups. Frequently, different ethnicities are underrepresented in research either because researchers do not expend the effort to include them or because the groups themselves distrust researchers and refuse to participate. Genetic data on gene frequency in diverse populations and the function of genes in different environments are critical to undertaking genome editing effectively and safely. Without the inclusion of diverse populations in research repositories, many groups will be excluded from or even harmed by genome editing because of lack of information.

The use of technology is not just if it excludes the impoverished and vulnerable who need help. The instruction *Dignitas personae* views scientific research with "hope" and desires that Christians will participate in the "progress of biomedicine." The instruction outlines the parameters to measure progress: "[The Church] hopes moreover that the results of such research may also be made available in areas of the world that are poor and afflicted by disease, so that those who are most in need will receive humanitarian assistance. Finally, the Church seeks to draw near to every human being who is suffering, whether in body or in spirit, in order to bring not only comfort, but also light and hope." [17]

Genetic Enhancement and Eugenics

As discussed above, the Catholic Church endorses strictly therapeutic interventions meant to correct harmful genetic mutations to heal disease,

17. CDF, *Dignitas personae*, n. 3.

provided such interventions are conducted morally and directed to human well-being. In contrast, genetic enhancement has a different purpose. While therapeutic modifications restore a patient to health, enhancement entails the alteration of genes to improve genetic traits beyond what is considered normal in a healthy person. The goal of enhancement intervention is to depart from what is naturally occurring in the human genome to boost such traits as strength, longevity, intelligence, height, and so on. Sometimes the distinction between therapy and enhancement is readily apparent. Sometimes an alteration does both. For example, consider genome editing to increase the height of a short-statured person from 3'4" to 5'4" or even 6'4." At what point does therapy become enhancement? Or consider increasing the intelligence of a child with the consent of the parent. Is that always unfair, given that he or she will probably have opportunities for education and employment that others will not? What if he or she grows up and discovers a cure for Alzheimer's disease or an environmentally safe energy source that addresses poverty in developing nations? Where and how will the Church and society draw the line between those interventions that truly advance human flourishing and those that exacerbate inequality and discrimination? Who will draw that line? These are difficult questions that remain unaddressed.

John Paul II uses this distinction between therapy and enhancement to provide guidance on the morality of enhancement in his 1983 address. He approves of enhancement as morally acceptable if it "improves the biological condition" and meets two standards: "Intervention must not infringe on the origin of human life ... [and] must avoid manipulations that tend to modify genetic inheritance and to create groups of different men at the risk of causing new cases of marginalization in society."[18] He proceeded to state that genetic interventions "should not flow from a racist and materialist mentality." It is scientifically possible that certain genetic enhancements could truly benefit individuals and societies while safeguarding the origins of human life and the integrity of the human person. John Paul II calls for an approach that will require exceptional wisdom and humility on the part of scientists and Church leaders.

These ethical concerns are very pertinent today, as scientific and technical progress makes enhancement nearly inevitable. There is widespread adoption of biomedically enhancing interventions that are

---

18. John Paul II, Address to the World Medical Association, n. 6.

currently available, such as cosmetic surgery, performance-enhancing drugs, exercise regimes, nutritional supplements, and so on. Much time and money are expended on bodily improvements, indicating that genetic enhancement will be readily adopted once it is deemed safe and effective. Individual choices of biomedical enhancements are usually influenced by societal and cultural norms which can change as cultural trends fluctuate. In contrast, genetic modifications are probably irreversible and cannot be altered to adapt to changing mores. For that reason and those discussed above, even if the moral conditions are met, genetic enhancements will be particularly challenging to evaluate ethically and biologically. It will be difficult, if not impossible, to foresee all the detrimental social consequences of personally beneficial enhancements.

Advances in genetic information and technologies like genome editing may raise renewed interest in eugenic practices or programs. The term *eugenics* stems from the Greek word for "good birth." It is an attempt to improve human beings through the inheritance of desired traits in one's offspring. Eugenics is an idea as ancient as the philosopher Plato and as recent as unethical governmental research in Germany and the United States in the 1990s. Genome editing reinvigorates the possibility of creating and selecting desirable offspring designed to fit individual preference and rejecting those deemed undesirable. The reasons why eugenics is unethical and immoral are too numerous for this discussion.[19] The connection of the abuses of human dignity which eugenics entails with genome editing could thwart the development of the potential benefits promised by this technology. Additionally, the thought that scientists' newfound and modest understanding of genetics will be able to design safe and beneficial improvements to human beings is probably hubris.

Using Genome Editing with Humility and Prudence

Developments in human genome editing catapulted these ethical issues into the forefront of science and bioethics. In 2023, only three years after the invention of CRISPR, the United States approved the use of CRISPR

---

19. Kevin FitzGerald, "Human Genome Editing: A Catholic Perspective," *National Catholic Bioethics Quarterly* 17.1 (Spring 2017): 107, doi: 10.5840 /ncbq20171719.

gene therapy to treat beta thalassemia and sickle cell anemia. These two serious and rare diseases are inherited disorders caused by a defective gene involved in red blood cell shape and function, a gene which is normally active only during fetal development. The treatment makes use of CRISPR to cut out the defective gene in the patient's own bone marrow cells, allowing the edited cells to repopulate the body and produce hemoglobin and normal red blood cells. At the time of this writing, the treatment is in its early stages and is considered curative.

This is a hopeful advance for patients suffering from two diseases for which treatments were not previously available. Yet all the risks of CRISPR discussed above still prevail: off-target effects, consequences which are difficult to predict, unethical applications, and extremely high costs. That said, for these two life-threatening diseases, detailed scientific and ethical analysis deemed the benefits sufficient to outweigh the risks. Continuing research on CRISPR to treat disease should inform decisions about clinical applications such as these and others, but only wisdom and good judgment will appraise and choose the applications of CRISPR that truly advance human flourishing.

When the Lord appeared to King Solomon in a dream at Gideon and said, "Ask what I shall give you," the new king responded humbly. Solomon described his shortcomings in leadership and asked, "Give your servant therefore an understanding mind to govern your people, that I may discern between good and evil, for who is able to govern this your great people?" (1 Kings 3:5–9). The Lord was pleased with his request and gave the king wisdom. If those entrusted with leadership and authority, as well as lay Catholics, approach the oversight of this new technology with humility and, like Solomon, ask the Lord for wisdom and judgment, God will have compassion and teach his people. In closing, "our impending power to alter our genetic heritage, coupled with a limited ability to predict the consequences of those alterations, cries out for a cautious and humble approach."[20]

---

20. Marilyn E. Coors, "Genetic Screening, Testing, and Engineering," in *Bioethics across the Lifespan*, ed. Marilyn E. Coors (Philadelphia: National Catholic Bioethics Center, 2015), 140.

4

LGBTQ+, the Normativity of Marriage, and Catholic Teaching

E. Christian Brugger

Catholic teaching today faces the great challenge of replying to misconceptions about human sexual identity advanced by LGBTQ+ proponents, ideas I will refer to here as the *new gender ideologies*.[1] Fundamental questions posed by these ideologies—questions to which this chapter replies—include: Does the embodied nature of human beings have any intrinsic significance for human identity? Are sex and gender dimorphic, expressed in and normalized by the biological facts of maleness and femaleness? Is there a fundamental alignment between the realities of maleness and femaleness and morally upright sexual behavior? Are the categories of man and woman socially constructed, sculpted like pieces of art by cultural forces and opening pathways to a wide range of alternative sexual identities and behaviors?

This chapter considers common ideas *both* about sexual orientation and sexual behavior as well as about so-called gender identity. *Sexual orientation* refers to one's tendencies of erotic attraction, to the groups or

---

1. See Human Rights Campaign, "Glossary of Terms," updated May 31, 2023, https://www.hrc.org/resources/glossary-of-terms. The acronym LGBTQ+ refers to lesbian, gay, bisexual, transgender, queer (or questioning), with "a '+' sign to recognize the limitless sexual orientations and gender identities used by members of our community." I use the plural *ideologies*, because despite common elements, there are considerable differences between the ideas of gender theorists.

individuals *toward* which one feels drawn romantically, emotionally, and sexually. *Gender identity* refers to one's inner feelings of and convictions about being a purported sex or gender either consistent or inconsistent with one's biological sex.

It is important to note at the outset that, although this chapter is framed as a critical response from the perspective of Catholic teaching, the Catholic response claims to be entirely consistent with right reason. This chapter, therefore, is offered not merely as a sectarian response to current pressing problems but as an account of what is true, of what is necessary for understanding what is good and right for human beings.

The new gender ideologies vary somewhat in the way they see the relationship between sex and gender. They agree that gender is a socially constructed reality;[2] that although male and female are natural biological realities, they are the "raw material," as one author puts it, "on which culture and society can do their work";[3] and that gender is "the result of that work, the social significance we invest in sex."[4] Gender is not physical, is not binary, has no innate alignment with biological sex, and has no

---

2. Arguably the most prominent gender theorist writing today is Judith Butler; see her most influential work, first published in 1990: *Gender Trouble: Feminism and the Subversion of Identity* (New York: Routledge, 2007).

3. Alex Byrne, "Is Sex Socially Constructed?," *Medium*, November 30, 2018, https://medium.com/arc-digital/is-sex-socially-constructed-81cf3ef79f07. Remarkably, some theorists even deny the fixity of biology: "Like the self the body can no longer be taken as a fixed—a physiological entity. ... The body itself has become emancipated—the condition of its reflexive restructuring. ... The body has become fully available to be 'worked upon' by the influences of high modernity. As a result of these processes, its boundaries have altered. It has, as it were, a thoroughly permeable 'outer layer' through which the reflexive project of the self and externally formed abstract systems routinely enter." Anthony Giddens, *Modernity and Self-Identity: Self and Society in the Late Modern Age* (Stanford, CA: Stanford University Press, 1991), 217–218. In rare instances, people are born with an anomalous condition known as intersex, possessing characteristics of both sexes. The rare intersex person should not be equated with persons identifying themselves as transgender, whose dimorphic biological features distinguish them unambiguously as males or females.

4. Byrne, "Is Sex Socially Constructed?"

inherent moral alignment with upright sexual behavior. Nature gives us male and female, and gender is the cultural meaning we construct out of them.[5] According to the new gender ideologies, gender expressions are as diverse as are people.[6] For purposes of this chapter, anyone who experiences or chooses to identify with a gender not corresponding to his biological sex is called *transgender*.

In responding to gender questions, Catholic teaching has a twofold challenge: first, to reply with sensitivity and mercy to gender-confused individuals who frequently suffer greatly and, second, to teach unambiguously the truths about sex, gender, and marriage. In other words, the Church must teach *veritas in caritate* (the truth in love). It is undeniable that a growing number of people today feel an incongruence between their sexed bodies and their gender identity. Some, for example, who are male feel—in some deep sense—female and, thereby, as though their bodies ought to look and be treated as female. If they experience severe psychological distress from this felt incongruence, they are said to suffer from what the American Psychiatric Association refers to as *gender dysphoria*.[7] Others do not report suffering distress. Both groups, however, experience a persistent unease about their sex and are tempted to undertake measures to alienate themselves from their bodies, to "transition," as they call it, away from their biological sex. This might take the form of acting, dressing, and wishing to be acknowledged as genders other than the one that corresponds to their sex. Or it might take more radical expressions in medical interventions, including hormone therapy and surgical procedures,

---

5. See Sarah Ditum, "What Is Gender, Anyway?," *New Statesman*, May 16, 2016, https://www.newstatesman.com/politics/2016/05/what-is-gender-anyway.

6. Emily Becker et al., "20 Common Gender Identity Terms as Defined by Psychologists and Sex Experts," *Women's Health*, internal quotation marks omitted, updated December 15, 2023, https://www.womenshealthmag .com/relationships/a36395721/gender-identity-list/. "Gender is a spectrum, and there is no finite number of gender identities. In fact, there are infinite places you can land on."

7. See American Psychiatric Association, "Gender Dysphoria," in *Diagnostic and Statistical Manual of Mental Disorders*, 5th ed., text rev. (Arlington, VA: APA, 2022), doi: 10.1176/appi.books.9780890425787.x14_Gender _Dysophoria.

meant to bring their bodies into closer alignment with what they feel is their true identity.

How Did We Get Here?

One might look around today and say, "What the heck is going on?" How did we get to a place where we celebrate the homosexual lifestyle with parades and dedicatory months, and where a large part of our country is agnostic as to whether biological sex has any relevance for personal identity? Although the intellectual and cultural dynamics leading to the present situation have been underway for nearly a century, relatively recent events have made it seem like the transition has happened overnight.

One of the most significant events was President Barack Obama's coming out as supportive of gay marriage in May 2012.[8] This contributed to a cascade of social effects. In June 2013, the US Supreme Court in *United States v. Windsor* ruled that the Defense of Marriage Act was unconstitutional.[9] In June 2015, the US military announced that its equal opportunity policy had been modified to include gay and lesbian service members.[10] The same year, Olympic gold medalist Bruce Jenner was featured dressed like a woman on *Vanity Fair* magazine and boldly

---

8. Rick Klein, "Obama: 'I Think Same-Sex Couples Should Be Able to Get Married,'" ABC News, May 9, 2012, https://abcnews.go.com/blogs/politics /2012/05/obama-comes-out-i-think-same-sex-couples-should-be-able-to -get-married. A year earlier, Obama had directed the US Department of Justice to cease defending the Defense of Marriage Act. AP / Huffington Post, "Obama: DOMA Unconstitutional, DOJ Should Stop Defending in Court, *HuffPost*, updated May 25, 2011, https://www.huffpost.com/entry /obama-doma-unconstitutioal_n_827134.

9. United States v. Windsor, 570 U.S 744 (2013); Ryan J. Reilly and Sabrina Siddiqui, "Supreme Court DOMA Decision Rules Federal Same-Sex Marriage Ban Unconstitutional," *HuffPost*, June 26, 2013, https://www.huffpost.com /entry/supreme-court-doma-decision_n_3454811.

10. Cheryl Pellerin, "DoD Updates Equal Opportunity Policy to Include Sexual Orientation," DOD News, June 9, 2015, https://www.defense.gov/News /News-Stories/Article/Article/604797/. See also Megan Slack, "From the Archives: The End of Don't Ask, Don't Tell," Obama White House, September 20, 2012, https://obamawhitehouse.archives.gov/blog/2012/09/20 /archives-end-dont-ask-dont-tell. In September 2011, the military abolished its "Don't Ask, Don't Tell" policy.

announced in an ABC interview with Dianne Sawyer: "Yes, for all intents and purposes, I am a woman." The US president publicly praised Jenner, saying his decision showed "tremendous courage."[11] Obama also was the first president to say *lesbian, bisexual,* and *transgender* in a State of the Union address.[12]

In June of that year, the Supreme Court in *Obergefell v. Hodges* created a right to homosexual marriage in all fifty states.[13] In May 2016, the US Department of Justice and the US Department of Education issued a directive forcing schools to provide students who identify as transgender with locker rooms and bathrooms of their choice.[14] In 2018 a man claiming to be a transgender woman was reported as being the first known case of a male breastfeeding a baby.[15] In 2019 the first biologically male athlete competed in an NCAA Division I women's cross country event.[16] In June 2020, the Supreme Court in *Bostock v. Clayton County* found that sexual orientation and gender identity are protected categories for employment law purposes, and Title VII of the Civil Rights Act of 1964 now prohibits

11. Buzz Bissinger, "Caitlyn Jenner: The Full Story," *Vanity Fair*, July 2015, https://www.vanityfair.com/hollywood/2015/06/caitlyn-jenner-bruce-cover-annie-leibovitz; ABC News, "Caitlyn Jenner Opens Up to Diane Sawyer," *Good Morning America*, 1:08, April 21, 2017, https://abcnews.go.com/GMA/video/caitlyn-jenner-opens-diane-sawyer-46926948; and Nick Gass, "Obama: Caitlyn Jenner Has Shown 'Tremendous Courage,'" *Politico*, June 2, 2015, https://www.politico.com/story/2015/06/barack-obama-responds-caitlyn-jenner-transgender-twitter-118551.
12. Alexandra Jaffe, "Obama Makes Historic 'Transgender' Reference in SOTU," CNN, updated January 20, 2015, https://www.cnn.com/2015/01/20/politics/obama-transgender-sotu/index.html.
13. Obergefell v. Hodges, 576 U.S. 644 (2015).
14. Caitlin Emma, "Obama Administration Releases Directive on Transgender Rights to School Bathrooms," *Politico*, May 12, 2016, https://www.politico.com/story/2016/05/obama-administration-title-ix-transgender-student-rights-223149.
15. Tamar Reisman and Zil Goldstein, "Case Report: Induced Lactation in a Transgender Woman," *Transgender Health* 3.1 (2018): 24–26, doi: 10.1089/trgh.2017.0044.
16. "How Did Transgender Runner June Eastwood Do in Her NCAA Division 1 College Debut?," LetsRun, September 3, 2019, https://www.letsrun.com/news/2019/09/how-did-transgender-runner-june-eastwood-do-in-her-ncaa-division-1-college-debut/.

employment discrimination on the basis of these categories.[17] In 2022 swimmer Lia Thomas became the first male athlete to win an NCAA Division I national championship in a woman's sport.[18] The list of milestones in the past decade could be greatly multiplied.

Until the twentieth century, the meaning of *gender* had little to do with social, psychological, or cultural aspects of human beings. Going back to the fourteenth and fifteenth centuries, it ordinarily meant kind or class or genus and was a word for classifying things, including persons, that shared common traits. More frequently it was a grammatical classification of nouns and pronouns (masculine, feminine, neuter) distinguished by the modifications they require in words grammatically associated with them. It was also a way of classifying humans according to their biological sex. Here gender was defined as the state of being male or female.

During the 1930s and 1940s, anthropologist Margaret Mead, in her studies on primitive peoples, began to emphasize what she referred to as the culturally influenced expressions of sex roles. She claimed that different expressions were "artificially assigned as masculine or feminine."[19] Commenting on this, Prudence Allen says that "Mead's conclusion about the relativism of sex roles and sex identities flowed over into a reflection on the word 'gender' itself." In one place, Mead asks the reader "to imagine, for instance, what a language could be like that had thirteen genders." Allen writes, "In her framing of this hypothetical question, Margaret Mead set the world stage, perhaps unknowingly, for a mutation of gender ideology to begin."[20]

17. Bostock v. Clayton County, No. 17-1618, 590 U.S. ___ (2020).
18. Katie Barnes, "Amid Protests, Penn Swimmer Lia Thomas Becomes First Known Transgender Athlete to Win Division I National Championship," ESPN, March 17, 2022, https://www.espn.com/college-sports/story/_/id/33529775/.
19. Margaret Mead, *Male and Female: A Study of the Sexes in a Changing World* (New York: William Morrow and Company, 1975), 373.
20. Mary Prudence Allen, "Gender Reality," *Solidarity: The Journal of Catholic Social Thought and Secular Ethics* 4.1 (April 2014): 6, 7, citing Mead, *Male and Female*, 13.

In the 1950s, psychologist John Money, following Mead, began to distinguish between sex as a biological reality and gender as a sex-based social role, a set of socially learned rules that a culture associates with biological sex (e.g., boys play with trucks, girls with dolls).[21] From the 1950s to the 1970s, feminist theory developed Money's idea. It began to argue that human nature is essentially genderless (i.e., we begin free of sex-based social roles) and that all social distinctions based upon sex are socially constructed. Around this time, a seminal piece of modern feminist literature, *The Second Sex*, was published by French writer Simone de Beauvoir. There she asserted that our consciousness of sexual difference is an artifact of culture. She famously stated, "One is not born, but rather becomes, a woman" (i.e., there is no essence of womanhood).[22] Only when we see the gap between biology and identity—between sex and the *I*—she argued, does it make sense to bring in the concept of gender to explain the experiences, roles, and socially imposed norms of sexuality.

In the 1980s, gay and lesbian studies was conceived as a university discipline; this was followed in the 1990s by queer studies. The latter, commonly referred to today as LGBT studies (e.g., at Yale and Berkeley), draws on critical materials from both feminist and gay and lesbian studies. From feminism it adopts the criticism of the concept of gender as pertaining to the essential self. From gay and lesbian studies, it adopts a harsh criticism of the historical understanding of the concept of sexual deviance, especially as the term was traditionally conceived through the lens of Christian moral teaching.

As noted above, the notion of gender as socially constructed is the central premise of the new gender ideologies. The apparent coherence

---

21. See John Money, *Gendermaps: Social Constructionism, Feminism, and Sexosophical History* (New York: Continuum International Publishing Group, 1995), 19. Money said that, late in her life, Mead encouraged him to continue his work breaking sexual taboos. See Allen, "Gender Reality," 8.

22. Simone de Beauvoir, *The Second Sex*, trans. Constance Borde and Sheila Malovany-Chevallier (New York: Vintage Books, 2011), 283. "Woman," she says, is a reflection of "what humanity has made of the human female" (48). For an excellent critique of de Beauvior's gender ideas, see Margaret H. McCarthy, "Gender Ideology and the Humanum," *Communio* 43.2 (Summer 2016): 278–281.

between sex, gender, and sexuality—for example, between maleness, masculine gender, and heterosexual desire—is culturally constructed (i.e., a product of culture, not nature). It arises over time through the repetition of socially sanctioned acts that have become ritualized such that they establish the appearance of an essential, ontological core gender.

The aim of the new gender ideologies is to deconstruct conventional sexual categories through shock and offense, and to replace them with an understanding of sexuality that emphasizes the shifting boundaries in sexual preferences, the uncertainties rather than clarity in gender identity, and the dominant influence of environment in conditioning sexual opinions. The categories of the familiar, the accepted, the normal, the decent, the moral, and the pure are all offspring of establishment narratives—that is, settled, socially sanctioned moral attitudes of the way things should be, constructed by those who occupy positions of power in the community and serving as the repositories of injustice, prejudice, narrowness, and exclusion. Just as the aim of postmodernist art is to shock, to produce outrage, to shatter the familiar, the aim of the queer movement is to queer: to render normal sexuality as strange and unsettling as possible, to challenge those who maintain that opposite-sex attraction is natural and that the categories of sex and gender are inherently binary, and to promote the concept of non-straightness, challenging all dominance of straight thinking. (The term *queer* can be used as an adjective, noun, or verb. Here it is being used as a verb, an action word.)

To promote these new gender ideologies socially, theorists speak about the imperative *to break the silence*, to encourage *coming out*. Those who have been locked *in the closet* are forced by cultural factors to remain silent.[23] Their silence reinforces the ignorance of the majority, who find it expedient to remain ignorant in order to perpetuate their power over sexual nonconformists. They think they know; hence, their ignorance is to them a kind of perverted knowledge, and this knowledge is their power. The silence of nonheterosexual and nonbinary people reinforces and perpetuates the repressive status quo.

---

23. For a seminal work of queer studies using the metaphor of the closet as its dominant framework, see Eve Kosofsky Sedgwick, *Epistemology of the Closet* (Berkeley, CA: University of California Press, 1990).

Critique of New Gender Ideologies

Positive Elements

Before we criticize the new gender ideologies—indeed, before we criticize the ideas of anybody—we should first ask what positive elements can be found in them. Although these ideologies advance some grievous errors, we can, nevertheless, draw some useful conclusions from what they emphasize. First, they draw needed attention to persons who experience sexual and gender confusion: to their humanity, sufferings, and needs. As stated above, it is undeniable that a not insignificant number of people feel uncomfortable with their biological sex as well as experience different sexual desires. Historically these populations have been misunderstood, ignored, and frequently rejected, including by members of the Christian community. They deserve appropriate attention, understanding, and—when they are open to receiving it—compassionate care; and every expression of unjust discrimination should be firmly rejected.

A further positive element, arising from the influence of feminism, has been to draw attention to "the values of femininity."[24] Although the concepts of woman and the feminine in the new gender ideologies are frequently unsound, indeed, radically so, when rightly conceived, they are critical for a balanced understanding of human life; and an appropriate contribution of woman and the feminine are essential for social and ecclesial health. We also can become sensitized to the dangers of binary thinking—us/them, in/out, for us / against us, friend/enemy—and to the need to emphasize grey areas and shifting boundaries, even though gender ideologies take these emphases to erroneous extremes.

Finally, the use of the metaphor of the closet can draw attention to problems of social censorship in the first half of the twentieth century when dealing with and speaking about sex and sexuality in daily

---

24. Congregation for Catholic Education, *Male and Female He Created Them: Towards a Path of Dialogue on the Question of Gender Theory in Education* (Vatican City: Vatican Press, 2019), nn. 15, 17; see also *Catechism of the Catholic Church*, 2nd ed. (Washington, DC: US Conference of Catholic Bishops / Libreria Editrice Vaticana, 2018 update), n. 2358. All subsequent citations appear in the text.

life. The failure to speak freely on these topics was particularly evident among parents and their children, seminary faculty and those in priestly formation, priests and the faithful, and teachers and their pupils. This censorship served to amplify the discourse it avoided and no doubt contributed to a more repressed psychology of the closet. We would do well to see the responsibility that our Church's own pastoral failures played in paving the way for the triumph of the sexual revolution. These failures frequently impeded the development of a rich and healthy understanding of sexuality among the Catholic faithful. Pope St. John Paul II's Theology of the Body has been an important step in appropriately breaking taboos related to the topic of sexuality in a way consistent with Christian faith and morals.

Errors

It is also important to understand the errors of the new gender ideologies. I will focus on two.

DUALISTIC ANTHROPOLOGY

The new gender ideologies hold what is called a dualist anthropology or understanding of the human person. Before we define dualism, let us be clear on the traditional Judeo-Christian anthropology. The human person is made up of a material element, the physical body, and a nonmaterial element, the spiritual soul. Together they form a human being. They do not exist as two separate natures. Rather, their union forms a single, human nature. Both body and soul are integral to—constitutive of—the *person*, establishing a unity so close that Catholic philosophy refers to the soul as the form of the body. The *Catechism of the Catholic Church* puts it this way: "The unity of soul and body is so profound that one has to consider the soul to be the 'form' of the body: i.e., it is because of its spiritual soul that the body made of matter becomes a living, human body; spirit and matter, in man, are not two natures united, but rather their union forms a single nature" (n. 365).

In their integrated unity of body and soul, humans are persons. Their whole being, spiritual and material, is personal. This is crucially important for understanding the central error of the new gender ideologies. According to Catholic thinking, not just the soul, not just the inner spiritual self, not just the psyche, not just the conscious subject, *but the body itself, too, is essentially and intrinsically personal.* Our biological life, our body, is invested with the full value of the person.[25] It is, therefore, correct to say both that "I *am* my body" and that "I *am* my soul."

According to the dualist conception, the human person is not an integrated unity of body and soul. Rather, the body is an instrument of the soul, of the inner spiritual self, of the conscious subject—an instrument of the person so conceived. As a canvas is to a painter, or a ship to its captain, so bodies are to the conscious self. Bodies are not intrinsically meaningful, but sub-personal, to be *used* as instruments of self-creation and self-actualization. Their meaning is imparted to them by how we use them. To the dualist, "*I am not* my body. I am only my soul (my consciousness, my inner spiritual self)."

The new gender ideologies are radically dualistic. They deny that bodies are intrinsically meaningful, personal, and normative for human identity—that my body tells me both my sexual identity and my gender identity. They assert that man and woman are socially constructed realities, that the alignment between maleness, masculine gender (and femaleness and feminine gender), and heterosexual desire is nothing more than a created narrative—and a harmful one at that—a repository for injustice, prejudice, and exclusion. The male and female bodies are nothing more than the "raw material on which culture and society can do their work." These views are opposed to the basic truth of our nature as made in the image of God, who created every person male or female. This truth grounds the teaching of the *Catechism* that "everyone, man and woman, should acknowledge and accept his sexual *identity*" (n. 2333, emphasis original; see also n. 2331).

If by nature I am male or female, then my sex and my gender, if not identical, are correlative. (Traditionally, *sex* and *gender* have been understood to be synonyms.) I follow here Christopher Tollefsen's view—which is consistent with but not specifically advanced in Catholic teaching—that gender is an aspect of human personality displayed to others, "adopted and shaped with a view to communicating some truth or falsehood about

---

25. Patrick Lee and Robert P. George, *Body-Self Dualism in Contemporary Ethics and Politics* (Cambridge, UK: Cambridge University Press, 2007), 1.

oneself."[26] In this sense, gender is not essential like biological sex. But although not essential, it is still correlative to my sex: rightly understood, my sex implies my gender. Their relatedness exists in the truths that gender communicates. Gender communicates truths (or falsehoods) *about* one's sex, in particular, about "one's embrace or rejection of the orientation towards the one form of the marital good (husband or wife), and one form of parenting (father or mother), that one's sex makes possible."[27]

In other words, gender communicates what I think about and how I act toward my sexed nature, a nature that makes possible my participation in marriage and parenthood. Males are disposed toward being husbands and fathers, females toward being wives and mothers. If I accept myself as male or female—as oriented in body toward being a husband and father or wife and mother—I communicate truths about my identity. If I reject these orientations, I communicate falsehoods. Gender, in this sense, speaks (as it were) the language of human identity, a language that can be true or false. Man and woman, therefore, are core genders aligned to the biological, bodily lives of males and females. This is surely part of what John Paul II meant when he repeated the maxim "The body reveals man" (i.e., the person).[28]

This conception is in no way incompatible with affirming that psychological and personality traits of men and women do not have any rigid appearance, but overlap and differ in expressions and degrees.[29] Some

---

26. Christopher O. Tollefsen, "Gender Identity," *Public Discourse*, July 14, 2015, https://www.thepublicdiscourse.com/2015/07/15308/.
27. Tollefsen, "Gender Identity."
28. John Paul II, general audience, Vatican City, November 14, 1979.
29. To say that expressions exist on a spectrum is not to say that maleness and femaleness are on a spectrum. Biological sex is a binary reality. On the one hand, this reality is genotypical (i.e., grounded in genetics): a pair of XY chromosomes representing maleness or a pair of XX chromosomes representing femaleness are found expressed in every one of the thirty trillion cells of the human body. On the other hand, it is also expressed phenotypically: males and females possess physiological features orienting them for a reproductive function, a function they perform jointly with another human being. Features include primary sex characteristics present at birth, the external and internal genitalia: the male penis and testes, the female

men are more nurturing, and some women are more aggressive; some boys like to play with dolls, and girls with trucks and guns. This does not imply that such persons *are* girls trapped in boys' bodies or boys trapped in girls' bodies. Manhood and masculinity express *truth* about a male person, although he might have certain characteristics commonly associated with women. As Tollefsen says, we must be careful not to frame too narrowly what the external communication of maleness and femaleness *should* look like, "such that some particular and closely drawn stereotype of masculinity or femininity has a strong normative claim. There are many ways of being masculine and feminine."[30]

Rejection of Traditional Marriage and Sexual Ethics

By rejecting the intrinsic value of differentiated male and female human bodies, and by affirming people in gender expressions that communicate falsehoods, the new gender ideologies deny the ontological complementarity of man and woman and, consequently, the normativity of the one-flesh procreative relationship of opposite-sex marriage that this complementarity makes possible. Genesis 1 and 2 teach not only that God created humans as male and female but that He created man and woman *for* each other. Human sexual differentiation is *for* marriage. The *Catechism* teaches, "Physical, moral, and spiritual *difference* and *complementarity* are oriented toward the goods of marriage and the flourishing of family life" (n. 2333, emphasis original). The new gender ideologies entirely reject the discourse of complementarity.

Although partners who undertake measures to alienate themselves from their biological sex can be committed to each other, as can same-sex partners, they cannot love each other *as* spouses. For spousal love—married love—is paradigmatically expressed in the complementary sexual union of husband and wife, a union that forms, for purposes of procreation, a single—one-flesh—biological system. That union, *Humanae vitae*

---

vagina, uterus, and ovaries. People also possess secondary sex characteristics that develop during puberty: female pubic hair, breasts, hormone levels, and broadened and more curvy hips; male pubic hair, muscle growth, vocal cord change, and formation of an Adam's apple.

30. Tollefsen, "Gender Identity."

teaches, possesses a two-fold meaning: unitive and procreative.[31] A biblically consistent view of sex and gender understands that man and woman were endowed from creation with a natural inclination for marriage and procreation, as John Paul II writes in his Theology of the Body: "In the mystery of creation ... man was endowed with a deep unity between what is, humanly and through the body, male in him and what is, equally humanly and through the body, female in him. On all this, right from the beginning, the blessing of fertility descended, linked with human procreation (cf. Gen. 1:28)."[32]

Noncomplementary sexual behaviors neither actualize a true union of bodies nor open the partners to conceiving new life; they are neither unitive nor procreative. Indeed, there is an intrinsic relationship between unity and procreation, for a true one-flesh union is defined not by a mere juxtaposition of body parts or by engaging with another person or persons in any mere sexual act, but by acts that are *per se* suited to bringing forth new life. Hence, the Church teaches that all sexual acts other than those performed in a human way between husband and wife and open to procreation are nonmarital and so illicit.[33]

Moreover, Vatican II teaches that through his sexed body, his "bodily composition," man "gathers to himself the elements of the material world; thus they reach their crown through him, and through him raise their voice in free praise of the Creator." Human sexual differentiation and complementarity are good, and what they make possible for men and women, namely, spousehood and parenthood, are good. "For this reason," the Council admonishes, "man is not allowed to despise his bodily life, rather he is obliged to regard his body as good and honorable since God has created it and will raise it up on the last day."[34] Gender

---

31. Paul VI, *Humanae vitae* (July 25, 1968), n. 12. The *Catechism* teaches that the union achieves a "twofold end": "the good of the spouses themselves and the transmission of life" (n. 2363).
32. John Paul II, general audience, November 14, 1979.
33. See Code of Canon Law, can. 1061 §1; and Congregation for the Doctrine of the Faith (CDF), *Persona humana* (December 29, 1975), n. 8. Referring to homosexual acts, the *Catechism* teaches, "They are contrary to the natural law. ... They do not proceed from a genuine affective and sexual complementarity. Under no circumstances can they be approved" (n. 2357).
34. Vatican Council II, *Gaudium et spes* (December 7, 1965), n. 14.

identities and sexual orientations that do not affirm the intrinsic goodness of the sexed body and the complementarity of man and woman are
at odds with genuine possibilities for marriage and procreation.

Pastoral Considerations

Although the Church reaffirms the essential anthropological complementary of human sexual identity and the moral normativity of properly
marital sexual acts, she also teaches that those who suffer from confusion
about their sexual inclinations and gender identities possess personal
dignity and should be treated in ways commensurate with that dignity.
The Church must be diligent to provide pastoral care, especially to assist
them to discern and live out the unique and unrepeatable role to which
God calls them in carrying out his divine plan. This *personal vocation*
extends to the whole of their lives, and the Church needs to assist them to
accept and reverence—regard as good and hold in honor—their embodied personal selves. Many may experience this goal as a heavy cross, especially during these times of sexual confusion.[35]

Likewise, pastoral ministers should not presume that people, even
people in their own congregations, know that all interventions aimed at
alienating oneself from one's body and all nonmarital sexual actions are
wrong.[36] Given today's widespread religious ignorance, powerfully secular currents of thought, and ubiquitously poisonous anti-Christian views
on sex and gender, the culpability for wrongful acts of all persons should

---

35. See Germain Grisez and Russell Shaw, *Personal Vocation: God Calls Everyone by Name* (Huntington, IN: Our Sunday Visitor, 2003), 35; and Vatican II, *Gaudium et spes*, n. 14. See also John Paul II, *Pastores dabo vobis*
(March 15, 1992), n. 39: "The word of God enlightens believers to appreciate
life as a response to God's call and leads them to embrace in faith the gift of
a *personal vocation*" (emphasis added).

36. For a rough formulation of the teaching against interventions aimed at
changing one's gender, see US Conference of Catholic Bishops Committee
on Doctrine, *Doctrinal Note on the Moral Limits to Technological Manipulation of the Human Body* (March 20, 2023), nn. 16–18. See also Dicastery
for the Doctrine of the Faith, *Dignitas infinita* (April 8, 2024), nn. 55–60,
esp. n. 60.

be assessed with care and judged with prudence.[37] But even acknowledging that culpability for sins can be mitigated by invincible ignorance and psychological distress, relativizing the truth cannot help another along the path of conversion and union with Christ. As Bishop Thomas Olmsted wisely teaches, "Our silence ... could reinforce that mistaken notion" that the Church accepts any "sexual activity outside of marriage."[38]

If persons we know engage in these harmful behaviors, we should assist them to come to peace with their sexed bodies, "look for an opportunity to invite them back to the faithful practice of a life of abstinence, assure them of the power of God's mercy to forgive and to bring fresh hope, and pray for their conversion."[39] It can be easy, amidst the confusions and controversies generated by gender debates, to lose sight of the fact that serious decisions concerning human sexuality always have relevance for salvation. God has blessed the human person with the great dignity of being able to cooperate freely with grace. This implies that it is possible to choose freely *not* to cooperate. For although we can never be certain that the subjective conditions for mortal sin have been fulfilled by another—and we should not judge—we are also unable to know that they have *not* sinned. And the worst pastoral response to those who have gravely sinned is to leave them in the state of alienation from God—to fail to help them receive the forgiveness of the Lord, who wishes to set them back upon the path to salvation. At the heart of the Church's pastoral response, therefore, is the call to repentance.

Teaching *veritas in caritate* about sex and gender is important not only for the salvation of individuals but also for the entire salvific mission of the Church. As Bishop Michael Burbidge explains, "So much of our faith rests on the natural truths of the human person, the body/soul unity, and the complementarity of man and woman. Jesus our Redeemer, the Son of God, assumes the body/soul unity of our human nature, sacrifices Himself and nourishes us by His Body, and is worshipped as the

---

37. CDF, *Letter to the Bishops of the Catholic Church on the Pastoral Care of Homosexual Persons* (October 1, 1986), n. 8.
38. Thomas J. Olmsted, "The Blessing of a Chaste Life: The Pastoral Care of Homosexual Persons," May 6, 2004, https://www.catholicsun.org/2013/06/26/the-blessing-of-a-chaste-life-the-call-to-holiness-of-homosexual-persons/.
39. Olmsted, "Pastoral Care of Homosexual Persons."

Bridegroom of the Church. The rejection of core natural truths regarding our humanity damages the 'template' that God uses to reveal Himself to us and to manifest His salvific plan for us."[40]

Anyone takes a risk today by defending and promoting the Catholic teaching that only sexual identities that express the truth of the sexed body and only sexual behaviors consistent with the goods of marriage conduce to integral human flourishing. They risk being called a homophobe or bigot or, worse, being cancelled, that is, subjected to what David Carlin calls "metaphorical lynchings."[41] It is becoming more and more common for opponents of Catholic teaching to be unwilling to engage the arguments of those who disagree and simply to assume that they are "haters."

Moreover, there is growing pressure to accommodate the convictions of the new gender ideologies not only by remaining silent in our disagreement but also by using language that implies agreement—for example, by using people's preferred pronouns, even when those pronouns contradict the person's biological sex.

We should resist these pressures for four reasons. To refer to a biological male using feminine pronouns, or a biological female using masculine pronouns, implies that we believe a male can become a female or a female a male. But these things are impossible. Thus, to imply that they are in fact possible is a kind of dishonesty. Moreover, to use false pronouns can be scandalous in the strict sense (i.e., it can be an enticement to sin) since, at very least, it reinforces people in false beliefs and may encourage them to make immoral choices. It also gives the appearance that we support the new gender ideologies, which can strengthen their proponents and discourage those who hold true views of sex and gender. Finally, to use false pronouns is a failure of Christian charity in the name of a kind of spurious compassion. The Gospels teach that we should assist the suffering with mercy (Luke 10:25–37). But reinforcing people in dangerous illusions that frequently lead them to undertake irreparably harmful measures is no more merciful than reinforcing an anorexic girl in the illusion that she is fat, thus supporting her inclinations to starve herself.

---

40. Michael Burbidge, *A Catechesis on the Human Person and Gender Ideology* (Arlington, VA: Diocese of Arlington, 2023), 10–11.
41. David Carlin, "The Dissenting Voice within Us," *Catholic Thing*, August 18, 2023, https://www.thecatholicthing.org/2023/08/18/the-dissenting-voice-within-us/.

If societal acceptance, or even just passive toleration, of the ideas of the new gender ideologies continues to grow much stronger, defenders of traditional marriage ("the beginning and basis of human society") and the family ("the first and vital cell of society") will wither to a remnant.[42] Subsequent centuries will look back on this time in history as the beginning of a new cultural dark age. And many souls will be lost.

But this is the time in which we live, our *kairos*,[43] the moment in history in which God's providence has placed us. And so, we can be sure that God will supply all the grace we need to accomplish his will, which surely includes the honorable effort of establishing genuinely Christian communal alternatives that protect and promote the truth that "sexuality is ordered to the conjugal love of man and woman" (*Catechism*, n. 2360).

---

42. Vatican Council II, *Apostolicam actuositatem* (November 18, 1965), n. 11; and John Paul II, *Familiaris consortio* (November 22, 1981), n. 42.

43. See Henry George Liddell and Robert Scott, *A Greek-English Lexicon*, rev. Henry Stuart Jones (Oxford: Clarendon Press, 1940), s.v. "kairos." *Kairos* signifies a time of great importance, a right, critical, and opportune moment for action.

5

Relativism and Toleration

Edward J. Furton

At the heart of relativism "is the right to define one's own concept of existence, of meaning, of the universe, and of the mystery of human life." This rephrasing of what Justice Antonin Scalia derisively labeled the "sweet-mystery-of-life passage" from Justice Anthony Kennedy's opinion in *Planned Parenthood v. Casey* requires the replacement of only a single word: *relativism* for *liberty*. Although Kennedy's words are a very poor description of liberty, they are a very good description of relativism. Relativism is the belief that all of us have the power to redefine experience, from its simplest aspects to its most complex, and thus create our own version of reality.

How did Kennedy mistake liberty for relativism? Liberty certainly gives us the freedom to be wrong, which is perhaps the best way to make sense of Kennedy's words, but it would be difficult to find any definition of liberty in the history of political thought that matches his description. Traditional liberalism defines the word positively as freedom of action. Negatively, it means freedom from oppression or restraint. Given these standard descriptions, it is obvious that liberty is limited in various ways. We are not free to mentally reconstruct the world. We cannot, for example, reconceptualize ourselves as creatures who are able to find happiness in isolation from others. We are social creatures. Neither can we live without food or warm clothing. Kennedy's phrasing suggests no such limitations. He implies that we need only think that something is so, and it becomes true.

Not only is liberty confined by physical constraints, but it is also bound by moral constraints. Hopefully, these are set by our own conscience, but in the absence of that guide, they must be safeguarded by public legislation and the enforcement of the law. True liberty always exists within a context of restraint, both physical and moral. We cannot intentionally harm others without committing wrong, no matter how liberating it may feel. If we are somehow able to escape responsibility for wrongdoing, we nonetheless deserve to be punished. Liberty has no power to set aside or ignore the moral law; it cannot turn something that is evil into what is good. These are obvious points, but the relativist either denies or cannot see them.

But let us take Kennedy at his word and examine his statement philosophically. How does one define one's own concept of existence? The word *existence*, of course, refers to what is—that is, to whatever exists or has being. Nonexistence refers to what is not. Any change in the current definition of the word *existence*, therefore, must necessarily signify what is not. Why? Because beyond what exists, all that remains as a possible referent for that word is that which is not. There *is* nothing else. If existence refers to being—and it does—then any change in its meaning must necessarily refer to what does not have being. I see no way around this simple observation.

Consider another word: *universe.* What does it mean to say that one has the right to define one's own concept of the universe? Here again the statement is contradictory. The universe is the totality of what exists—that is, the word signifies a highly complex system of matter and fundamental forces that science has, for centuries, attempted to fully understand. Any redefinition of the concept *universe*, therefore, necessarily describes something that the universe is not. I am free to redefine the universe as something that is not subject to the law of gravity, but the fact remains that no such world exists. We could go through the remaining terms in Kennedy's sweet-mystery-of-life passage with the same result. The problem of referring to what is not affects the whole, which leads to the obvious question, Was Kennedy implicitly signaling to us that he knew the conclusion he offered was false?

Probably not. That would require some level of epistemological self-awareness. For the relativist, the meaning of concepts does not derive from our experience of the world but from the mind's construction of a counter world. Thus, a concept can contradict nature and still be true. The word *male* can refer to a person who is physically female, and the word *female* can refer to a person who is physically male. The falsity of these descriptions is not a mark against them, but proof that we can redefine reality. Unfortunately, the disassociation of words and meanings has real-world consequences. As a result of relativizing the terms *male* and *female*, many people have suffered life-altering injuries, including children. A boy's concept that he is a girl, no matter how strongly he thinks it is true, will never overcome the physical disfigurements that result from so-called gender-affirming care.

The Objective Guidance of Nature

Kennedy's relativistic conclusion about liberty in *Casey* has had wide-ranging effects on American jurisprudence and culture. *Obergefell v. Hodges* concerned marriage. The question before the Court was whether heterosexual and homosexual unions could equally reflect that ancient institution. In the past, marriage had been defined as the life-long union of a man and a woman. Why? For the simple reason that men and women are naturally suited to sexual union. This is a biological fact. Homosexuals, in contrast, cannot have children. Men can acquire ova, use them in in vitro fertilization, and have one or more embryos implanted in a surrogate, but their union is sterile. Similarly, women can acquire sperm for in vitro fertilization, though in this case, they could provide the ovum and carry the child. But the fact remains that their union is sterile. This is a natural limitation on our freedom. *Obergefell* pretends to set these natural limitations aside. *Marriage*, like the words *existence* and *universe*, need not refer to something that actually exists. Marriage can mean the sexual union of couples who cannot have children.

Relativism appears to widen the meaning of truth, but in fact it narrows it by erasing differences. The following are some examples: In the general category of cultural relativism, no one culture can be described as superior to another. Thus, in politics the modern form of government known as the democratic republic is no better or worse than the monarchical form of the Middle Ages. Their apparent difference is merely a matter of perspective. In economic theory, feudalism is no better or worse than capitalism. Servitude to the land is no better or worse than the modern hourly wage system. In food production, specialized agricultural machinery is no better or worse than the use of hand tools and plough horses. For the relativist, there is no objective criterion that can decide which option is better in any of these comparisons. The order of nature is not a guide to judgment for the relativist but is, instead, an obstacle to the redefinition of truth.

Generally, when we want to know what a thing is, we examine it, understand its function, and classify it as a type within some larger class. Aristotle defines *human being* as a rational animal. We belong to the genus animal, and our specific difference is rationality. Despite the progress made in the sciences, this definition remains as serviceable as it was when it was first set down. If there are no distinguishing marks in nature that can separate one thing from another, definition becomes impossible. This is not a defect for the relativist but an avenue for redefining words and meanings. He does not want objective definitions. He denies the existence of distinguishing marks, because their existence limits his freedom to construct new worlds. The relativist wants to break free of natural restraints. Relativism, finally, is a rebellion against nature.

To deny nature as the standard of truth is to privatize the world so that each of us dwells within a realm that is fundamentally disconnected from that of everyone else. Fortunately, no one truly believes this, not even the relativist. Even after affirming that relativism is true, the relativist lives as if it were not. He works with others within a common world, uses language with agreed-upon meanings, and inhabits a political order whose rules, laws, and customs are followed by most everyone. None of this would be possible if relativism were actually true. What, therefore, are we to make of the obviously contradictory stance of relativism? Is the relativist unaware that even those who profess it do not believe it? Just as Kennedy's sweet-mystery-of-life passage is so absurd that it suggests he might be signaling to us that even he obviously knows it is false, so too is the absurdity of relativism so extreme that it is hard to believe that anyone accepts it at face value. Perhaps no one does.

This suggests that relativism is not a theory about the truth but, instead, an argumentative strategy. For those who wish to advance a cause, especially a very controversial cause such as homosexual marriage, the claim that we can redefine reality allows one to ignore the obvious contradictions presented by nature. Heterosexual and homosexual marriage, as mere social constructs, do not have the type of distinctive natural features that enable us to distinguish them. The same is true of socially constructed ideas of male and female. A man can be a woman and a woman can be a man, because the order of nature is irrelevant. Relativism is not a theory about the truth but a strategy for advancing ideas that do not conform to the order of nature. The relativist ignores, dismisses, and seeks to overthrow nature. Nature, as the standard for the truth, is a stumbling block to his arguments and an obstacle to his goals.

But this leads to a paradox, for at the same time that he argues that there is no objective truth, the relativist also claims that his own arguments are true. He claims, for example, that one can change his or her sexual identity by subjective intention. Indeed, he is passionate about this claim and defends it with great energy. But given that he holds that we cannot know the truth, how can he assert that his own views are true? Put differently, if all claims of knowledge are relative, why should his particular view take precedence over that of others? For those who are not relativists, the answer is easy. Truth is what corresponds to nature. A man has certain distinctive biological features, and a woman has others. So, to what does the relativist appeal as the standard of truth? Here we discover his totalitarian tendencies. If the natural world is not the guide to judgment, then disputes about truth must be settled by force. With nature banished, no other criterion is available. Whoever has the power to compel another to assent to his opinion, therefore, possesses the truth.

In a relativistic world, force becomes the standard, because there is no criterion to which reason can turn. Reason is effectively neutered. What is called truth about homosexual marriage, therefore, is settled by whomever has the power to compel others to submit. Truth is imposed. Those who refuse to conform to the truth must be brought to heel by force. Thus, we saw that the initial appeals for the toleration of homosexual marriage were offered on the grounds that all should be free to love whoever they please. When the Supreme Court ruled in favor of this view, there followed the persecution of those who continued to hold that marriage has its true foundation in nature. The dissenters to the Court's opinion expressed their moral objections in trivial ways, such as the unwillingness to make baked goods or the denial of venues for homosexual weddings. These refusals were met with outrage, condemnation, and lawsuits. Force substituted for reason, because truth for the relativist is the power of the stronger.

Abuse of Toleration

Toleration is not a Christian virtue, but it is a positive good that merits the support of civil society. Strong advocacy for toleration began during the Protestant Reformation when the doctrinal disputes among Christian denominations led to vicious persecutions and religious warfare. Figures like John Locke recommended that Christians live in peace with each other despite differences over doctrine. The toleration of error was preferable to dissension and hatred. The defenders of toleration also believed that each person should be free to affirm only what he truly believes. No one should be compelled to assent to what he thinks is false. But toleration is not relativism. To tolerate is not to agree with what one believes to be in error. Neither does it require a blanket denial of objective truth. A tolerant person judges that others hold erroneous views but chooses to live with them peaceably. Tolerant people hope for agreement in the future.

Toleration is attractive to Christians, who are called to forgo harsh judgments and to show compassion toward others. Are we not obliged to overlook others' faults? Yes, that is true, but the relativist wants others to show respect for what is not true. That is quite different. This demand does not derive from the virtue of toleration but from the desire to gain an advantage. Once respect for falsehood is granted, the relativist uses force to compel conformity. Those who are tolerant, in contrast, do not use force to compel. They live with differences. Moreover, they recognize that the application of force is a violation of conscience, which the virtue of toleration seeks to prevent. Neither does the relativist hold out any hope for arriving at possible future agreements. Christians should be on guard against appeals to toleration because they are often rhetorical strategies designed to gain a foothold that can later be used against dissenters.

One common tactic is to misinterpret Matthew 7:2, where Jesus tells his followers not to judge: "For as you judge, so will you be judged, and the measure with which you measure will be measured out to you." This is a reformulation of the Golden Rule. We should treat others as we would like to be treated, which also means that we must judge ourselves as we judge others. If my judgment of you is harsh or unfair, then I should expect others to judge me in a similar manner. This does not mean, however, that we should avoid making judgments altogether, as if we were to abandon our conscience. We must always be careful to distinguish between good and evil, and this involves judgments concerning both ourselves and others. Christ did not come to set aside the Ten Commandments but to complete and perfect them. The commandments are a summary of the natural law whose general governing principle is that we should pursue what is good and avoid what is evil. We cannot follow this rule unless we make judgments.

What Jesus opposes in Matthew 7 is hypocrisy. We must take the plank out of our own eye before noticing the speck in others'. But avoiding hypocritical judgments does not mean shutting down our natural ability to distinguish right and wrong. There is nothing hypocritical in stating that a thief, an adulterer, or a murderer does what is wrong. Neither is it hypocritical to state that homosexual marriage is contrary to the order of nature. This is, instead, an observation of the centrality of sexual union to the married state. Neither is it immoral to fault those who destroy healthy organs through gender-affirming therapy. Jesus did not oppose judgments, even harsh ones, if they were true. He did not hesitate, for example, to call the Pharisees whitewashed tombs. Neither did he ask us to forgive those who have not hurt us but have hurt others. Only those who have suffered injury can grant pardon. I have no power to grant forgiveness to someone who has injured you.

Given his influence, St. Paul is sometimes called the second founder of Christianity. His travels are recorded by St. Luke in the Acts of the Apostles, which is followed by Paul's letters. He was certainly not afraid to judge. In his letter to the Romans, he says, "Hate what is evil; cling to what is good" (12:9). Hate is a very strong word, but he uses it. In philosophical terms, what is hated cannot be made an object of love, because the two are opposites. Evil actions are an appropriate object of our hatred. We *should* hate what is evil. Of course, we must distinguish between the sin and the sinner, but indifference to wrongdoing is a serious mistake, because it allows serious harms to continue, thus permitting further suffering and making it possible for others to be hurt. Here are some actions that are proper objects of hatred: murder, rape, incest, cruelty, treason, betrayal, and similar wrongs. We certainly should not approach such things with indifference. Strong contempt for evil is necessary to motivate the concerted action needed for its prevention and elimination.

The claim that Jesus taught us not to make judgments is an effective tool of relativists against Christians and causes some to foolishly tolerate evil. The phrase "Do not judge, lest ye be judged" is quoted as if it were divine support for the philosophy of relativism. Who are you to make judgments? I thought you were a Christian. Have you not heard that Jesus tells us not to judge others? Presumably the true Christian is one who passes through life without differentiating between right and wrong, good and evil, or virtue and vice. Perhaps he is permitted to judge his own actions, but judgments about others are forbidden. Thus, the teachings of Jesus are made to fit the cramped views of the modern relativist. And how is it that the relativist has acquired the authority to interpret Christianity for Christians? He rejects objective truth, and this includes truth itself. In his condemnation of Christians for making judgments about homosexual marriage, transgender surgery, abortion, and other moral evils, the relativist judges others and contradicts his own assertions about Christ's teaching.

Natural Purposes and the Objective Good

In the debate over the meaning of truth, the relativist seems to have the easier argument. He denies objectivity and so has little incentive to engage in debate. He need only sit back and object to what his opponent is saying. One can assert that the relativist's view is false, but he will respond that this confirms his opinion that truth depends on one's perspective. You have your truth, I have mine. The defender of objectivity, in contrast, must show that the notions of true and false depend on some external standard. This is more difficult. One can offer the theory that truth depends on a correspondence between the mind and reality, but how does one identify the existence of goods and evils? The sun and rain are obviously external, but good and evil do not seem to have the same type of objective presence. Where, exactly, are they? How can one show that these are objects in nature no less than sun and rain?

The argument is not as difficult as it might seem. Let *good* be the achievement of some end in nature. Let *evil* be the failure to achieve that goal. If this is the right starting point, then good and evil are objective, because they are connected to natural purposefulness. When we look closely at nature, we find that everything in nature does indeed have a purpose that can be identified; for example, all living things seek to preserve themselves in existence. Consider a simple plant, such as a tree. Every part of the tree is ordered to self-preservation. The roots draw up water. The bark protects the trunk. The leaves reach out for sunlight. The tree is an assemblage of purposes that serves a much larger purpose: that of preserving life. The tree also sets seeds and releases them to propagate its species. This too is on behalf of life. The failure to remain rooted, to preserve its trunk, or to synthesize sunlight because of disease, lack of space, or some other debilitating factor—all of these are evil, because they destroy the life of the tree and its power to generate its kind.

The reflective person can see that nature exists as a teleological order. Things seek to fulfill their purposes. To understand what is good for human beings, therefore, we need to identify the purposes that are natural to us. Securing them will enable us to enjoy what best fulfills us as human beings. Of course, we need what any other animal needs to survive, such as food and shelter, but we can enjoy higher purposes, such as knowledge, conversation, and friendship. These goods fulfill our nature in a way that cannot be experienced by any other creature, because they require the power of reason. Every rational creature takes delight in them—or should. A man without friends may have great wealth, but he cannot be truly happy. To live without friends, conversation, or knowledge would produce a shallow and empty life. We can, therefore, also answer the second part of the relativist's objection. These goods have an objective existence that can be quantified. That quantity may not be as obvious as rain or sunshine, but it is measurable. Some people have more of these goods, others less. Some people have more (or better) friends, enjoy more (or better) conversations, and have acquired more (or better) knowledge.

In response, the relativist might say that good and evil, unlike rain or sunshine, are not physical and, therefore, do not exist objectively. He thus reverts to his position that good and evil are mental constructs. Ask a scientist if he can detect the difference between good and evil, and he will say no. A scientist has no instruments of a type that would be able to identify such things. He can measure rainfall by using a simple gauge, but good and evil do not register on his instruments, no matter how sensitive. To be real, the relativist may contend, a thing must have some basis in matter and so present us with some sort of physical appearance. Good and evil are not like that. They are not material things. Therefore, they must be creations of the mind. Truth depends on the perspective of the viewer.

The reply to this reasoning is that there is indeed evidence to show that good and evil do have an existence in matter, though we must also note that they are not reducible to matter. An eye that has lost its ability to see differs materially from one that retains its sight. Any physician can identify the difference. The natural purpose of the eye is to see, and the loss of that purpose is an objective evil. Moreover, good vision has an objective measure: 20/20. Will the relativist say that whether one can see is just a matter of perspective? We can agree that vision is not merely material, but is instead a perfection of the eye, and so exists as something over and above its mere physical existence. An engineer might construct an exact replica of a human eye using material parts, but it would not be able to see unless it were incorporated into a living being who can experience the good of vision.

Those who recognize that there are purposes in nature have an advantage in life. They can adjust their conduct to better achieve what perfects human nature. Smoking is bad for one's health, so it can be abandoned. Exercise is good for health and so can become part of a weekly routine. Promiscuity spreads sexually transmitted diseases, a chaste life does not. Beyond the ability to make such basic improvements in life, the one who admits that nature is the standard for human conduct is also able to offer sound judgments on the goods of the larger social order. One such good is the family. For decades cultural elites have disparaged the family, saying that marriage is not essential to childrearing, that children can do just as well in cohabiting households, and that the sexual differences between men and women are irrelevant to family life. Yet the best predictor of success in life, especially for young men, is the presence of a father and a mother within the home.

This leads to a final observation. The constructs of family life imagined by the relativists do not produce good results. This is a fact. Despite this fact, the relativist sees no reason to adjust his opinions. He has closed his mind to objective truth and so cannot see that the purposes of nature are the true guide to human fulfillment. One who refuses to adjust to failure is truly an ideologue. So long as relativists dominate our culture, dismiss nature as a common standard, reject the objectivity of good and evil, construct their own truths, and compel others to assent to what is false, the possibility of social improvement will be beyond our grasp. Especially vulnerable will be the young, who will continue to be deprived of the encouragement they need to seek meaning in life through fulfilling the purposes that satisfy our human nature: the love between man and woman, the birth and rearing of children, and the blessings of a lifelong commitment to marriage.

6

Language and Its Power in Society
Elena Kraus, MD

Stop and consider the profound power of language. The words we use are foundational for our beliefs, attitudes, morality, and ultimately our view of reality. Historically, any major change in cultural attitudes and actions is preceded by a change in how an action or the object of our actions is considered and described in our minds and, subsequently, in spoken or written language. In the marketplace of thoughts entailed by pluralism, the currency is the language used to determine the value of ideas, bolstering the power of one group of people against another or twisting the meaning of contrary positions to subvert, ridicule, or bankrupt them. As William Brennan notes in his book *Dehumanizing the Vulnerable*, "Words can also act as a force for justice or a weapon of repression, an instrument of enlightenment or a source of darkness."[1]

Given the power of language, it is critical to be intentional about the words we use to map out our own paths of cultural engagement and change, taking particular care to resist the commandeering of our terminology by others. This chapter explores this power of language, as the foundation for civil discourse, to shape our view of the world, its effect on culture, and its weaponization for the benefit of social or political agendas. As a consequence, the necessity to preserve critical definitions and arguments to support the dignity of human life as a foundational ethical

---

1. William Brennan, *Dehumanizing the Vulnerable: When Word Games Take Lives* (Chicago: Loyola University Press, 1995), 1.

principle in our culture should become apparent. Equipped with an awareness of the ideological stakes involved in framing the debate with the words we use, the dignity of persons must be communicated and upheld as the bedrock of civil society.

The Words We Use Matter

The power of naming shapes culture. The words used to describe an action color its meaning, changing the perception and interpretation of its morality. Although we are taught that words cannot hurt us (but sticks and stones can), this is not true. Name-calling not only affects how we see ourselves and others but can foster a climate of antagonism. Although disparagement "does not always result in violence, it is invariably an essential component of any large-scale oppression: discrimination, segregation, enslavement, or annihilation."[2]

It is no wonder, then, that what it means to be human begins in the words we use to define a human, and issues of when and how life begins have historically been the source of much semantic argumentation. To be clear, when human life begins can be scientifically observed and described as the point at which a genetically distinct individual is formed. Generations of human biologic and embryologic research demonstrate that human life begins at conception, or fertilization. Irrevocably, at this point a new person (at that time called a zygote) is created with its own individual genetic makeup and programmed to develop into a mature human being like any one of us, given the proper environment. The form does change, but its nature does not.[3]

Despite the detailed scientific understanding of the minute-to-minute processes of early human development, and the websites and apps that track the progress for expectant mothers, there remains much debate concerning when precisely life begins (the definition of life) and the related moral and legal implications. This is apparent among

2. Brennan, *Dehumanizing the Vulnerable*, 3.
3. American College of Pediatricians, "When Human Life Begins," position statement, updated March 2017, https://acpeds.org/position-statements /when-human-life-begins; and Steven Andrew Jacobs, "The Scientific Consensus on When a Human's Life Begins," *Issues in Law and Medicine* 36.2 (Fall 2021): 221–233.

organized physician associations, particularly those concerned with women's health. These disputes usually are motivated by a desire to frame early human life such that various actions can be taken without certain moral implications rather than to answer the question accurately. The absence of public debate about when the lives of other mammals begin underscores this point. This authority to decide the matter clearly has grave social and political ramifications.

Although there may have been a time where the American College of Obstetricians and Gynecologists (ACOG) agreed that the point of fertilization, or conception, was the start of life, as far back as 1965, the organization has promoted a definition of pregnancy as beginning at the time of implantation.[4] Now ACOG and a long list of women's health associations accept this latter view. Note the shift of focus to pregnancy from the start of life, which is no longer clearly addressed. The word *life* as a defined phenomenon is avoided, and instead the term *pregnancy* is used, which is defined as "a physiologic state of a woman that follows implantation of a blastocyst(s)." ACOG further preempts those who would use conception as a critical point in human development, explicitly describing it as "a lay term that has no scientific validity and is not generally used in the medical literature because of its variable definition and connotation."[5] Notwithstanding this claim, the term is used even in more recent manuscripts published in ACOG's journal, which does not baulk at referring to what is removed in an abortion as "products of conception."[6] One can regularly find examples in other high-impact journals

---

4. American Congress of Obstetricians and Gynecologists (ACOG), *ACOG Terminology Bulletin: Terms Used in Reference to the Fetus* (Chicago: ACOG, 1965), cited in American College of Pediatricians, "When Human Life Begins."

5. ACOG, *Revitalize: Gynecology Data Definitions*, s.v. "pregnancy," updated November 19, 2018, https://www.acog.org/-/media/project/acog/acogorg /files/pdfs/publications/revitalize-gyn.pdf.

6. Baruch Feldman et al., "Obstetric and Perinatal Outcomes in Pregnancies Conceived after Preimplantation Genetic Testing for Monogenetic Diseases," *Obstetrics and Gynecology* 136.4 (October 2020): 782–791, doi: 10.1097 /AOG.0000000000004062; and Jenny S. George et al., "Utility of Office Hysteroscopy in Diagnosing Retained Products of Conception following Early Pregnancy Loss after in Vitro Fertilization," *Obstetrics and Gynecology* 142.5 (November 2023): 1019–1027, doi: 10.1097/AOG.0000000000005382.

where *conception* is used as a medical term that indicates the beginning of a pregnancy.[7]

The Ideology Behind Words

These propagated definitions are not accidental, but intentional and based in a well-established system of beliefs—that is, they have ideological foundations. They do not come from established facts or rational frameworks, but instead develop in service of an agenda. Truly, a small adjustment of focus, even from life to pregnancy—which has much less developed associations with humanity and personhood—allows a much wider breath of space to justify violent actions against the unborn. Furthermore, with this definition of pregnancy, contraception is defined as any "action taken to prevent pregnancy," and an abortifacient is "a substance intended to cause termination of a pregnancy so that it does not result in a live birth."[8] Therefore, "none of the FDA-approved contraceptive methods are abortifacients because they do not interfere with a pregnancy and are not effective after a fertilized egg has implanted successfully in the uterus."[9] The potential postfertilization effects of contraceptives that may prevent implantation of a formed embryo are then unimportant, as a pregnancy does not exist between fertilization and implantation.

ACOG has published an advisory document to guide discussions about abortion "to help inform language choice for those writing about reproductive health to use language that is medically appropriate, clinically accurate, and without bias." The document outlines how this language should describe a "fetal heartbeat" as "'embryonic cardiac activity' before eight weeks of gestation and 'fetal cardiac activity' after eight weeks of gestation" and to promote the term *uterus* in place of *womb*, as the latter "is a nonmedical term that can be used to apply an emotional value

7. Huiling Xu et al., "Pregnancy Weight Gain after Gastric Bypass or Sleeve Gastrectomy," *JAMA Network Open* 6.12 (December 2023), e2346228, doi: 10.1001/jamanetworkopen.2023.46228.
8. ACOG, *Revitalize*, s.v.v. "abortifacient," "contraception."
9. ACOG Committee on Health Care for Underserved Women, "Committee Opinion No. 615: Access to Contraception," *Obstetrics and Gynecology* 125.1 (January 2015): 251, doi: 10.1097/01.AOG.0000459866.14114.33.

to a human organ."[10] If the definitions and language were not important, ACOG and many other organizations such as Planned Parenthood and the American Civil Liberties Union would not make the effort to publish documents that dictate the definitions of words critical to their agenda and, furthermore, outline how one should use terms to talk about controversial entities like abortion.[11]

Ceding that life exists at conception or using language that indicates abortion is violent in any way weakens an agenda of unquestioned use of contraceptives and unrestricted access to abortion. The intentional way individuals and groups approach naming and defining critical entities in early human life enables them to avoid any resultant accountability to nuance, mislead medicine and the public, and justify the use of medications and actions that a reasonable person could argue threaten or end a human life. This keen interest in semantic framing can be seen in all corners of culture. For instance, medical definitions outlined by ACOG include defining an early zygote as a "cell" and abortions as procedures that "terminate a pregnancy."[12]

The National Security Agency published an internal document, which subsequently was leaked, that is "a glossary of terms and language commonly used in dialogue regarding diversity, equity, inclusion, and social justice to be used as a reference." The definitions are biased and based in a specific ideology, and they add more confusion than clarity to words, many of which were created for political correctness. A disclaimer states that "the meaning of these words may change and evolve," but the

---

10. ACOG, *ACOG Guide to Language and Abortion*, September 2023, https:// www.acog.org/-/media/project/acog/acogorg/files/pdfs/publications /abortion-language-guide.pdf.

11. Judy Gold et al., *How to Talk about Abortion: A Rights-Based Messaging Guide* (London: International Planned Parenthood Federation, 2015); and American Civil Liberties Union, "Your Mini Guide to Discussing Abortion Rights at the Dinner Table," ACLU, November 23, 2022, https://www.aclu .org/news/reproductive-freedom/your-mini-guide-discussing-abortion -rights-thanksgiving.

12. ACOG, *Revitalize*, s.v.v. "induced abortion," "zygote."

document is "a tool meant to build a shared language of understanding."[13] These references are more likely to build an unaccountable foundation that can be weaponized culturally and politically against those who do not adopt their use and meaning.

Regardless of scientific validity or accuracy, perpetuating specific semantics ultimately can and does have significant effects. Control of language facilitates control of thought. Indeed, "eventually semantic corruption leads to the adulteration of thought itself. ... Avoidance of the scientific fact, which everyone really knows, that human life begins at conception and separation of the idea of abortion from the idea of killing" are essential pillars of the campaign to gain widespread acceptance of violent acts against unborn humans.[14] Having these mischaracterizations accepted as truth also involves the active participation of prominent people and institutions.

How Words Translate to Actions

It is well studied and understood in health care that the words we use matter and can be associated with bias in how physicians practice medicine. These differences in practice may even contribute to health care disparities. Evaluation of physician documentation has shown patterns of expressing both positive and negative feelings toward patients, including "compliments, approval, and personalization" as well as "disapproval, discrediting, and stereotyping." Using stigmatizing and negative language to describe patients in the medical record has been shown to influence physician attitudes as well as prescribing behavior, such as reduced prescription of pain medications, and can affect the quality of care patients receive. The words used in health care do "more than transfer information between patients and healthcare providers—[they have] the potential to shape therapeutic

---

13. National Security Agency, *P65 DEI Glossary*, May 6, 2022, available in Spencer Lindquist, "Exclusive: Leaked NSA Doc Reveals Massive Woke Glossary Pushing Critical Race Theory, Gender Ideology at Intel Agency," Daily Wire, November 15, 2023, https://www.dailywire.com/newsexclusive -leaked-nsa-doc-reveals-massive-woke-glossary-pushing-critical-race -theory-gender-ideology-on-govt-employees.
14. Brennan, *Dehumanizing the Vulnerable*, 8, internal quotation marks omitted.

relationships … affect how patients view their health and illness, reflect healthcare workers' perceptions of their patients, and influence medical care and treatments offered."[15]

The words chosen to name and describe phenomena as significant as human life also pave the way for the ultimate treatment of these individuals. Brennan demonstrates how those in power have, throughout history, targeted and ultimately initiated violence against a person or group of people by first dehumanizing them through language of disparagement. Indeed, any potential target is "cast in such a negative or inconsequential light that whatever is done to them, no matter how horrendous, is considered perfectly justifiable."[16] He systematically illustrates how unborn babies and other victimized groups are described as animals, parasites, illnesses, inanimate objects, waste products, and ultimately nonpersons with no humanity and no rights. Although Brennan's book was published thirty years ago, these patterns are still observable today. Language is used to spread lies and false perceptions and to justify antagonism as the initial phase of warfare. The new truth that is proposed and received by a culture encouraged to be open to diverse ideas, philosophies, and values then paves the way for those in power to first think and then do significant evils against others.

Nowhere is this pattern expressed more clearly than in our cultural, social, and scientific battle against the unborn, which is, at its heart, a war against the dignity of the human person. The language used in this war is embedded in our cultural consciousness through its frequent and vehement propagation in the name of science, equality, and ethics. Although the unwanted unborn have been frequently reduced to a level below animals throughout history, of all words used to dehumanize them, the

---

15. Caitríona Cox and Zoë Fritz, "Presenting Complaint: Use of Language that Disempowers Patients," *BMJ* (April 2022), e066720, doi: 10.1136/bmj-2021-066720. See also Jenny Park et al., "Physician Use of Stigmatizing Language in Patient Medical Records," *JAMA Network Open* 4.7 (July 2021), e2117052, doi: 10.1001/jamanetworkopen.2021.17052; and Anna P. Goddu et al., "Do Words Matter? Stigmatizing Language and the Transmission of Bias in the Medical Record," *Journal of General Internal Medicine* 33.5 (May 2018): 685–691, doi: 10.1007/s11606-017-4289-2.

16. Brennan, *Dehumanizing the Vulnerable*, 3.

ubiquitous *fetus* portrays a more subhuman or even nonhuman entity than does *embryologic human*, *baby*, or *unborn child*. The words used generally imply whether the preborn human is wanted or not.[17] Indeed, in obstetrics and gynecology, pregnancy is not infrequently joked about as a sexually transmitted infection. Other recent descriptions refer to early pregnancy as "unfeeling cells" and propagate the belief that establishing the personhood of an early pregnancy is in direct contention to the personhood of women.[18]

Indeed, since *Dobbs v. Jackson Women's Health*, the next frontier of definition legislation is that of personhood laws, where unborn children are seen as persons that warrant legal protection and rights. Alternatively, the right to abortion can also be enshrined into state constitutions.[19] Although clear definitions of personhood are frequently avoided by those who support abortion, personhood laws are tenaciously opposed, as seeing a preborn human as having personhood and its associated rights threatens not only abortion but arguably various applications of reproductive endocrinology and contraception.[20] Even Justice Samuel Alito remarked in the majority opinion in *Dobbs*, "Our opinion is not based on any view about if and when prenatal life is entitled to any of the rights enjoyed after birth."[21] After the *Dobbs* decision, abortion was no longer federally protected, opening up argumentation on the definition of personhood and the significant implications for morality and legislation. ACOG published a statement on personhood explicitly opposing

> any proposals, laws, or policies that attempt to confer "personhood" to a fertilized egg, embryo, or fetus. These laws and

---

17. Brennan, *Dehumanizing the Vulnerable*, 78–79.
18. Sarah Jones, "Abortion Is Morally Good," *Intelligencer*, May 17, 2019, https://nymag.com/intelligencer/2019/05/theres-nothing-wrong-with-abortion.html.
19. Mary Ziegler, "The Next Step in the Anti-Abortion Playbook Is Becoming Clear," opinion, *New York Times*, August 31, 2022, https://www.nytimes.com/2022/08/31/opinion/abortion-fetal-personhood.html.
20. Madeleine Carlisle, "Fetal Personhood Laws Are a New Frontier in the Battle over Reproductive Rights," *Time Magazine*, June 28, 2022, https://time.com/6191886/fetal-personhood-laws-roe-abortion/.
21. Dobbs v. Jackson Women's Health Organization, 597, U.S. 215, 263 (2022), cited in Carlisle, "Fetal Personhood Laws."

policies are used to limit, restrict, or outright prohibit access to care for women and people seeking reproductive health care. … Assigning rights to fertilized eggs compromises access to essential facets of medical care. Elevating the legal status of fertilized eggs (embryos) to that of women and pregnant people has wide implications for access to medications, medical interventions, and management of high-risk pregnancies. … Requiring physicians to treat an egg, embryo, or fetus as a person with the same scope of rights as people in their care will jeopardize the lives and health of those patients. This conflicts with the patient-clinician relationship and contradicts fundamental, deeply rooted principles of medical ethics.[22]

In this way, ACOG takes an entity it has intentionally dehumanized and weighs it against the well-being of the mother, health, and ethics, thus paving the way to justify abortion in all forms and at all stages of development. In fact, it becomes a moral obligation to make abortion available to women as a fundamental right and critical medical procedure. Accordingly, a person intending to protect such an entity as an embryo will be viewed as ethically compromised and as disregarding women's rights, reproductive rights, and good health care.

There are many other examples in medicine of a change in definition being associated with an evolution in thought. The American Society of Reproductive Medicine formerly referred to in vitro fertilization with the sole purpose of have a boy or girl as sex selection. Published opinions from the ethics committee of the ASRM in 1999 discouraged this practice, citing issues of gender equality, a focus on inessential characteristics, the health risks of the procedure, and justice in use of medical resources.[23] Only two years later, the position changed to indicate that sex selection for the sole purpose of having a child of the opposite sex of existing children

---

22. ACOG, "ACOG Statement on 'Personhood' Measures," position statement, November 9, 2022, https://www.acog.org/clinical-information/policy-and-position-statements/position-statements/2022/acog-statement-on-personhood-measures.

23. Ethics Committee of the American Soceity of Reproductive Medicine (ASRM), "Sex Selection and Preimplantation Genetic Diagnosis," *Fertility and Sterility* 72.4 (October 1999): 595–598, doi: 10.1016/S0015-0282(99)00319-2.

may be less ethically problematic, but a provider is under no obligation to perform it.[24] Along with an increasing acceptance of the practice, a sub-category of sex selection termed *family balancing* was offered and then reaffirmed in 2022.[25] As ethical standards changed over time, how these actions are named also changed.

A similar evolution of thought can be seen in the stance of the American Medical Association to physician-assisted suicide, originally held to be antithetical to the principle of "first, do no harm" and expressly considered an unethical practice for physicians. The practice is still described as "fundamentally incompatible with the physician's role as healer" in the AMA *Code of Medical Ethics*.[26] The AMA maintained the same position on so-called medical aid in dying (MAID) until 2019, when the AMA Council on Ethical and Judicial Affairs indicated a possible softening of the organization's position, citing "the irreducible moral tension at stake for physicians with respect to participating in assisted suicide" and "the thoughtful moral basis for those who support assisted suicide."[27] Nevertheless, the term MAID is not found in the latest *Code of Medical Ethics*.

In November 2023, after a new petition regarding physician-assisted suicide suggested a more neutral stance, the AMA proceeded to change the official language to "medical aid in dying." A resulting informational report from the AMA concluded that the "AMA's policy of opposition to MAID is now arguably in conflict with its own code of ethics and requires

---

24. ASRM Ethics Committee, "Preconception Gender Selection for Nonmedical Reasons," *Fertility and Sterility* 75.5 (May 2001): 861–864, doi: 10.1016/S0015-0282(01)01756-3.

25. ASRM Ethics Committee, "Use of Reproductive Technology for Sex Selection for Nonmedical Reasons: An Ethics Committee Opinion," *Fertility and Sterility* 117.4 (April 2022): 720–726, doi: 10.1016/j.fertnstert.2021.12.024.

26. American Medical Association (AMA), "Physician-Assisted Suicide," opinion 5.7, *Code of Medical Ethics* (2016), http://www.ama-assn.org/.

27. AMA, *Report 2 of the Council on Ethical and Judicial Affairs (2-A-19)* (Chicago: AMA, 2019), 1; and Dallas R. Lawry, "Rethinking Medical Aid in Dying: What Does It Mean to 'Do No Harm'?," *Journal of the Advanced Practitioner in Oncology* 14.4 (May 2023): 309, doi: 10.6004/jadpro.2023.14.4.5.

re-examination."[28] Such changes are not unexpected. The AMA believes that the *Code of Medical Ethics* "sets ethical guidance to how physicians should interact with patients" and that "all physicians should uphold the ethical standards set forth in the *Code*."[29] However, the code is also described as a necessarily "living document," and the proposed ethical framework is "distinct from personal virtue or morality."[30] Supporting changes in our perceptions and actions requires changes in how we name and describe them.

Civil Engagement in Current Culture

The words we use and how we communicate are foundational to civil discourse. Recognizing the dignity of people and our own humanity in dialogue is fundamental to what it means to be human. Civil engagement is increasingly challenging, particularly for those with worldviews no longer considered mainstream. Current discourse is dominated by critical theory, feminism, and Marxism, characterized by narratives of the oppressors versus the oppressed. The oppressors generally are privileged, have ties to Christianity and capitalism, prefer limited government, and adhere to traditional concepts of gender, marriage, and family. If one can prove he or she is the most oppressed or victimized, he or she makes the rules, operating from a culture of fear and shame and without accountability.

The experience of public discourse seems much less civil, with shaming, word-policing, and gaslighting rampant, leading to confusion, fear, and silencing of those at odds with the accepted narratives. Engagement can be disorienting, with reality seemingly reversed, words redefined, and an overdeveloped sense of political correctness discrediting

---

28. AMA, *Informational Report A of the American Medical Association Resident and Fellow Section (I-23)* (Chicago: AMA, 2023), 10.

29. AMA, "FAQ," under "What is the AMA Code of Medical Ethics?," *Code of Medical Ethics*, accessed February 14, 2024, https://code-medical-ethics .ama-assn.org/faq.

30. AMA, "About," AMA Code of Medical Ethics, accessed February 14, 2024, https://code-medical-ethics.ama-assn.org/about; and AMA, "Code of Medical Ethics," AMA Code of Medical Ethics, accessed February 14, 2024, https:// code-medical-ethics.ama-assn.org/.

anyone who would step outside of the semantic boundaries created, no matter how illogical or incorrect they are. This is the so-called woke culture, which operates through an approach of intimidation and shaming while also remaining unaccountable to logic and clear definitions. In many circumstances, arguments do not even seem to matter, with conclusions foregone and reason falling by the wayside.

So, how is it possible to have respectful, rational conversations in our current culture? Such dialogue not only is an integral part of our humanity and relationship with others but will reveal important truths and protect the vulnerable. Engagement can be intimidating. Outing your ideas and beliefs can draw criticism and downright hostility. This pattern is regularly displayed in the mainstream media and academia when discussing politics, public health, and issues of social justice, further instilling a sense of fear and avoidance in sharing our ideas—ourselves—with others. The first step in becoming more comfortable and effective in these opportunities for good discussion is to understand certain common tactics, including straw man arguments, ad hominem attacks, and a lack of neatly defined terms. Then one can clearly set boundaries for what is an acceptable interaction, define terms, and intentionally expose divergence from good argumentation. With reason, zeal, and bravery, we can express the essential components of our argument with no apologies.

I recently had an experience testifying in support of a state bill making abortion illegal after a heartbeat was detected, allowing exceptions for rape and medical emergencies. It was ultimately associated with another bill limiting medical and surgical interventions for gender transitioning until after the age of nineteen. The testimonies and arguments I heard from senators and my fellow physicians were eye-opening. The way the good-faith language of medical exceptions was twisted to indicate that the bill was too restrictive but also too unclear, and that physicians had to worry about criminal liability when dealing with medical complexities, instilled confusion and fear. I observed competent physicians express how they would not be able to care for patients because of the fear of going to jail, something that had never even crossed my mind in my practice of medicine or in considering the limits of the bill. It was wrongly referred to as an abortion ban when there were clear exceptions for rape and threats to the health of the mother.

I believed I was trying to bring a rational, experienced medical view that would help protect unborn babies and protect children and teens from making life-altering decisions about hormonal and surgical treatment for gender dysphoria. Instead, a senator opposing the bill, with handwaving and emotion, described anyone who would support this bill as a killer of women and children who has blood on their hands. I was completely baffled, as I had used the exact same words to describe those who participate in abortion. Her words were compelling, but they reversed reality. Somehow the theoretical risk that a woman would die because she could not obtain an abortion (i.e., when the so-called treatment in the referenced situations is delivery, not a dilation and extraction per se) or that a child would commit suicide because he or she was unable to act on the desires for gender transition, became a reality that made me the murderer. Not once did the opposing testimony acknowledge that the unborn child's dignity and status as a life should, in any way, weigh in these considerations. If the life of the unborn child was even acknowledged, it was defined as a *pregnancy* or *fetus*, betraying their bias.

The reality was twisted to a place where abortion was the treatment for a multitude of life-threatening emergencies in pregnancy, including suicidality, and sex-change operations saved children's lives by healing their dysphoria and preventing suicide. These so-called facts were simply false. Still, those who put them forward are not held accountable by the culture or the media, and their reasoning remains unchallenged. Those who would question or oppose have their intelligence and character attacked, being branded as the oppressors of freedom, women's rights, and health and, ultimately, as the real murderers. Straw men surface everywhere—unsubstantiated claims about abortion bans, medical emergencies that can be treated only with dilation and extraction, and the potential treatments and outcomes for gender dysphoria—and are much easier to vilify and dispute than are the real arguments and the actual practice of medicine. In our culture, instead of an open, rational market of expression and ideas, alternative viewpoints are policed by those imposing radical agendas within the demands of political correctness. Unfortunately, most leading institutions of education, the arts, religion, law, philosophy, ethics, medicine, and politics are increasingly dominated by "a politically correct cultural elite bent on imposing its radical agenda onto every facet" of life.[31]

If one can identify the errors in reason and question the key definitions and tenets of opposing arguments kindly and clearly, he or she has already gone a long way toward healthy engagement and thoughtful expression of the truth. Another critical aspect of success is creating and maintaining boundaries regarding language and reasoning. You must establish clear limitations when engaging with those who disagree with you and who routinely miscategorize, misunderstand, and misrepresent your views. Do not apologize. Remain steadfast in your own definitions, resisting the temptation to bend or surrender the meanings you establish, especially if you think doing so would be incorrect or not in line with the truth. Explicitly question your opponent's assumptions. Pay close attention to how others name and define things.

Understanding language, its use, and its misuse is part of the challenge. If key nuances of language can be recognized, focused on, and not surrendered, even the act of clarifying the definitions of terms can be an instrument of engagement and argumentation. This can be done in a nonthreatening way simply by asking questions and expressing sincere interest. Ask for examples when statements you believe are baseless are made. Calmly correct when your words or ideas are misrepresented. Cling to the truth in both your own and your interlocutor's arguments.

Finally, we must provide an alternative, positive view of the primary points of argument, protecting core tenets from being altered or disregarded as part of a critical theory narrative. As Brennan argues, providing "positive, personalized, and exalted images of the victims as worthwhile human beings whose oppression can no longer be tolerated" is a foundation for the success of any true human rights movement, because, just like negative labels, these images have the power to create a profound change in how people are perceived and therefore treated.[32] In the realm of human dignity, it simply involves showing others the truth about the value of the human person in all stages, shapes, and abilities, using sound reason and scientific evidence. Indeed, "some of the most memorable portraits of the

---

31. Brennan, *Dehumanizing the Vulnerable*, 15.
32. Brennan, *Dehumanizing the Vulnerable*, 19.

preborn as genuine members of the human family have been etched by physicians and scientists" on the basis of their investigation and observation of the earliest stages of human life.[33] Conversely, we must use well-established natural law and science to reject alternative characterizations. Do not accept deceptive reasoning or compromise your position, even in attempts to engage with others who disagree with you.

Aleksandr Solzhenitsyn, in his essay "Live Not by Lies," released on the day he was arrested in 1974 before being exiled from his homeland of the Soviet Union to West Germany, urged individuals in his country to resist the Soviet ideology, the lies that were reshaping his society to the specifications of those in power:

> When violence bursts onto the peaceful human condition, its face is flush with self-assurance. ... But violence ages swiftly, a few years pass—and it is no longer sure of itself. To prop itself up, to appear decent, it will without fail call for its ally— Lies. For violence has nothing to cover itself with but lies, and lies can only persist through violence. ... And therein we find, neglected by us, the simplest, the most accessible key to our liberation: a *personal nonparticipation in lies!* ... For when people renounce lies, lies simply cease to exist.[34]

When engaging rationally with others, do not be afraid to call attention to the irrationality or error of arguments, and focus on one or two unwavering truths—truths like "all humans, from the point of fertilization, are unique beings who are deserving of dignity and respect and have a right to live." Question anyone who tries to define who has a right to live and who does not, which is, at its heart, elitist and discriminatory toward a defined group of people.[35] Work toward illustrating a human beauty so clear that it changes the perceptions of others.

What we call things significantly affects our perception of their goodness or lack thereof. If one pays attention, it is painfully obvious that

---

33. Brennan, *Dehumanizing the Vulnerable*, 206.
34. Aleksandr Solzhenitsyn, "Live Not by Lies," February 12, 1974, trans. Yermolai Solzhenitsyn, emphasis original, Alexandr Solzhenitsyn Center, https://www.solzhenitsyncenter.org/live-not-by-lies.
35. Brennan, *Dehumanizing the Vulnerable*, 199.

preserving or changing how we name things is used to illustrate particular realities and highlight acceptable actions in line with the agendas of those in power. The building blocks of language are the foundation for significant social, political, religious, and medical trends in our culture that ultimately lead acceptable behavior and morality. Engaging with these trends and discussing a variety of contentious topics is difficult, complicated, confusing, and even scary. We must have faith in our Church, our God, and ourselves. Our beliefs are supported by reason, science, charity, and the contemplation and argumentation of thousands of saints over two millennia.

Be brave, be bold, and your unapologetic expression of ideas will be seen and respected, even if you are not shown understanding and respect. Stand firm in your knowledge that you defend the dignity of the human person in all shapes and forms, a truth that transcends time, culture, and any current social, philosophical, religious, medical, and academic trends. May we use caution with language that supports lies and subverts the dignity of the human person or anything good, beautiful, and true. May we never cower when others twist our words into those of hate. May we use our words and ideas to affirm, encourage, support, and love each other.

7

Seven Christian Principles for Thriving with Artificial Intelligence

Christopher M. Reilly

In a very short time, artificial intelligence technology—the programming that enables computers and devices to calculate, analyze, and reason in ways similar to human beings—has emerged out of science fiction into reality, with the potential to radically transform our daily lives. It seems that AI will support an almost-infinite array of exciting applications, anything from rewriting essays in a particular style to discovering previously unimagined proteins for new medicines, seamlessly adding or removing items from images, intuitively managing the intake process at large hospitals, or enabling a stroke victim with a paralyzed leg to walk with "smart" pants.[1] It is not a stretch to imagine that nearly all aspects of human life will be affected in some way.

---

1. Benjamin Alexander Albert et al., "Deep Neural Networks Predict Class I Major Histocompatibility Complex Epitope Presentation and Transfer Learn Neoepitope Immunogenicity," *Nature Machine Intelligence* 5 (July 20, 2023): 861–872, doi: 10.1038/s42256-023-00694-6; Jessel Renolayan, "Kahun Integrates Its AI Clinical-Intake Tool with Tel Aviv Sourasky Medical Center," *Tech Times*, August 7, 2023, https://www.techtimes.com/articles/294809/20230807/; and Paul Pigott, "AI: Stroke Patient Helped to Walk by High-Tech Trousers," BBC News, August 14, 2023, https://www.bbc.com/news/uk-wales-66311632.

At the same time, there is great fear over the self-sufficiency, ruth-less pursuit of programmed goals, superior calculative intelligence, and lack of transparency in the theoretical and actual methods of AI systems and robots, so much so that even AI experts have difficulty explaining why AI models produce certain results. In recent surveys, 83 percent of Americans believe that "AI could accidentally cause a catastrophic event," nearly 70 percent say that "they are 'concerned' about artificial intelligence in healthcare," and 75 percent "have little trust to no trust" that AI com-panies will care for their well-being.[2] It is not surprising, then, that the roller coaster of existential anxiety and hopeful anticipation about AI can extend into Christians' thinking about religion, trust in God's plan, and confidence in their own consciences. How can anyone securely decide on the goodness of AI, let alone make moral decisions about applying it for entertainment, work, medicine, and other purposes?

While recognizing the immense value of the new technologies, Pope Francis expressed a number of concerns about AI on the 2024 World Day of Peace; anyone concerned about the effect of AI should read the doc-ument in its entirety. Francis stated that "developments such as machine learning or deep learning, raise questions that transcend the realms of technology and engineering, and have to do with the deeper under-standing of the meaning of human life, the construction of knowledge,

---

2. AI Policy Institute, "Poll Shows Overwhelming Concern about Risks from AI as New Institute Launches to Understand Public Opinion and Advo-cate for Responsible AI Policies," news release, accessed November 6, 2023, https://theaipi.org/poll-shows-overwhelming-concern-about-risks-from-ai-as-new-institute-launches-to-understand-public-opinion-and-advocate -for-responsible-ai-policies/; Katie Jennings and Alex Knapp, "Innova-tionRx: 70% Of U.S. Adults 'Concerned' about AI In Healthcare," *Forbes*, August 9, 2023, https://www.forbes.com/sites/alexknapp/2023/08/09/in novationrx-70-of-us-adults-concerned-about-ai-in-healthcare; and Ipsos, "Americans Hold Mixed Opinions on AI and Fear Its Potential to Disrupt Society, Drive Misinformation," news release, May 4, 2023, https://www.ipsos .com/en-us/americans-hold-mixed-opinions-ai-and-fear-its-potential -disrupt-society-drive-misinformation.

and the capacity of the mind to attain truth."[3] Specifically, AI poses threats to pursuit of the common good, privacy, data ownership and intellectual property, transparency of decision-making, individual freedom of decision, recognition of the uniqueness of human persons, and peaceful resolution of international conflict. Further, AI can generate "discrimination, interference in elections, the rise of a surveillance society, digital exclusion and the exacerbation of an individualism increasingly disconnected from society." Virtuous living with AI requires both prudence and humility, a "sense of limit" in the way we develop and apply new technologies: "Recognizing and accepting our limits as creatures is an indispensable condition for reaching, or better, welcoming fulfilment as a gift."[4]

Francis also reminds us that there is plenty of room for hope and virtuous action in living with AI: "When human beings, 'with the aid of technology,' endeavour to make 'the earth a dwelling worthy of the whole human family,' they carry out God's plan and cooperate with his will to perfect creation and bring about peace among peoples."[5] By patiently listening to the wisdom found in the Bible and Church teachings, and with prayer, we can discover the answers we seek. Remember the words of Ecclesiastes 1:9: "What has been is what will be, and what has been done is what will be done; and there is nothing new under the sun." On this journey of understanding and evaluating the goodness of AI in our personal lives and society, let us keep our focus on the following seven principles:

1. The existence of the created world is good.

2. Human persons have a unique dignity and special purpose.

3. Technology and its use are good when they contribute to true human development.

4. Artificial products and tools are morally neutral in themselves but parts of a larger moral context.

---

3. Francis, *Artificial Intelligence and Peace*, message for the 57th World Day of Peace (January 1, 2024), n. 3.

4. Francis, *Artificial Intelligence and Peace*, nn. 3, 4.

5. Francis, *Artificial Intelligence and Peace*, n. 1, citing Vatican Council II, *Gaudium et spes* (December 7, 1965), n. 57.

5. The real structure of AI influences persons' welfare and habits of moral virtue.

6. The end of the world will develop in and through Christ.

7. We are called to faith and hope.

The Existence of the Created World Is Good

The first chapter of the book of Genesis tells us that, when God created the various parts and things of the world, He repeatedly saw that it was good. The followers of the true God have always known something revolutionary and joyful: God's very being is goodness; it just is who He is.[6] Everything that exists participates in that being by the will of God and so enjoys the divine goodness in a limited way.[7] This may sound very academic or theoretical, but the fundamental link between the goodness of creation and God's goodness is deeply ingrained in the minds of all who have faith in God, our Creator (*Catechism*, nn. 295–301).

Human persons, of course, also have a great aptitude for creativity. Machines and the technologies that run them, like AI, are the achievements of freely acting and thinking human beings. What we can never do, however, is create something out of nothing. Everything we make—whether it is a smartphone, a communications network of billions of machines (the internet), or a living being grown in a lab from certain types of cells—comes from the things that God provides. In our creative achievements, we have a great opportunity and a moral responsibility to be stewards, or caretakers, of God's good creation.[8] As Pope St. John Paul II said, "The believer, in a sense, is 'the shepherd of being,' that is, the one who leads all beings to God, inviting them to sing an 'alleluia' of praise."[9] This role of steward is very different from the current misguided desire to flee from the real world by creating a new virtual reality with the magic

6. *Catechism of the Catholic Church*, 2nd ed. (Washington, DC: US Conference of Catholic Bishops / Libreria Editrice Vaticana, 2018 update), n. 294. All subsequent citations appear in the text.
7. The philosophy behind participation in being was particularly advanced by St. Thomas Aquinas in the late medieval period. See, for example, *Summa theologiae* I.6.4.
8. Francis, *Laudato si'* (May 24, 2015), nn. 1–15.
9. John Paul II, general audience (Vatican City, January 17, 2001), n. 1.

of AI. In fact, there is no such thing as a virtual reality; consider that even the invisible electronics and computer codes of AI depend on huge, physical data centers, consume considerable amounts of energy and the natural resources that produce it, and require droves of human workers to design, monitor, and censor their output.[10]

Human Persons Have a
Unique Dignity and Special Purpose

It is crucial, when evaluating the moral goodness of AI, to remember that the human persons who create, use, and are affected by it have a dignity that is not shared by anything else in God's creation. This is not simply a special favor from God or a function of our achievements or capabilities, but is based in the very nature of the human person as having a spiritual soul combined with a physical body: "He alone is called to share, by knowledge and love, in God's own life. ... This is the fundamental reason for his dignity. ... Being in the image of God the human individual possesses the dignity of a person, who is not just something, but someone" (*Catechism*, nn. 356, 357). We are formed uniquely for our destiny to be in the presence of God; human nature and true human progress are inseparably linked.

The dramatic achievement of AI, and its powerful and rapidly growing ability to make machines appear to think or reason with sophistication, has inspired many people to imagine using AI to radically improve human beings by either directing our behaviors (sometimes secretly or forcibly) to be more productive or ethical, connecting our bodies and brains to computers or the internet, or granting an artificial immortality by electronically recording, storing, and imitating our thoughts and personalities.[11] Already some researchers have integrated human brain cells

---

10. See Niamh Rowe, "'It's Destroyed Me Completely': Kenyan Moderators Decry Toll of Training of AI Models," *The Guardian*, August 2, 2023, https://www .theguardian.com/technology/2023/aug/02/ai-chatbot-training-human -toll-content-moderator-meta-openai.
11. Vanessa Bates Ramirez, "Grief Tech Uses AI to Give You (and Your Loved Ones) Digital Immortality," Singularity Hub, August 16, 2023, https:// singularityhub.com/2023/08/16/grief-tech-uses-ai-to-give-you-and-your -loved-ones-digital-immortality/.

with computer chips that can communicate with the internet.[12] From a moral perspective, researchers and society must recognize that human beings can truly benefit only from our growth in Christian virtue and friendship with God, not from any supposed upgrade in our given nature as both souls and bodies. We are not only minds full of information that can be encoded electronically, nor are we merely biological beings that can be analyzed and manipulated by technicians and scientists without deep moral consequences.

It will also be important to avoid thinking of technology, which is only an artificial rearrangement of God's creation, as having its own destiny or laws of progress to which human beings must submit or conform. Pope St. Paul VI warned, "Every kind of progress is a two-edged sword. It is necessary if man is to grow as a human being; yet it can also enslave him, if he comes to regard it as the supreme good and cannot look beyond it."[13]

AI and the machines it governs, including robots that look and act like human beings, are never equivalent to human persons in any moral sense. Such a view is called anthropomorphism, and we need to be aware that we have a strong (maybe natural) tendency to interpret nonhuman things in this unrealistic way.[14] Complex AI systems will increasingly appear to have free will as they are designed to respond differently to new situations and even to alter their own governing algorithms in the face of success or failure, but they will always lack the full spontaneity and creative freedom of the human will, and they are designed and made by human beings out of the materials available in God's creation. The value and dignity of any AI-governed machine, then, will always be determined by how well it achieves the goals originally intended by the designers, even if this purpose is defined broadly to act as much as possible like a human person. The value and dignity of each human person, however, is

12. Zinnia Lee, "This AI Startup Wants to Be the Next Nvidia by Building Brain Cell–Powered Computers," *Forbes*, June 21, 2023, https://www.forbes.com /sites/zinnialee/2023/06/21/cortical-labs-brain-computer.

13. Paul VI, *Populorum progressio* (March 26, 1967), n. 19.

14. Elizabeth Broadbent, "Interactions with Robots: The Truths We Reveal about Ourselves," *Annual Review of Psychology* 68 (January 2017): 627–652, doi: 10.1146/annurev-psych-010416-043958.

in our nature and purpose, which are tied to our destiny of being in the presence of God (not only because we have consciousness, intelligence, logical reasoning skills, and so on).

Technology and Its Use Are Good When They Contribute to True Human Development

John Paul II encourages us to continue applying our minds, skills, imagination, and effort to developing new, productive technologies like AI as a part of true human development as children of God: "Work is a good thing for man—a good thing for his humanity—because through work man *not only transforms nature*, adapting it to his own needs, but he also *achieves fulfilment* as a human being and indeed, in a sense, becomes 'more a human being.'"[15]

Such technologies and their use, however, should be governed by our fundamental purpose as spiritual beings. As the Congregation for the Doctrine of the Faith teaches, "Science and technology are valuable resources for man when placed at his service and when they promote his integral development for the benefit of all; but they cannot of themselves show the meaning of existence and of human progress. Being ordered to man, who initiates and develops them, they draw from the person and his moral values the indication of their purpose and the awareness of their limits."[16] The Pontifical Academy for Life and leaders from Microsoft, IBM, Italy, and the United Nations signed a document in 2020 called the *Rome Call for AI Ethics*, which emphasizes "the development of an artificial intelligence that serves every person and humanity as a whole; that respects the dignity of the human person, so that every individual can benefit from the advances of technology; and that does not have as its sole goal greater profit or the gradual replacement of people in the workplace."[17]

There is, however, a certain structural tendency of AI to emphasize goals that are instrumental—that is, these systems are intended to select

---

15. John Paul II, *Laborem exercens* (September 14, 1981), n. 9, emphasis original.
16. Congregation for the Doctrine of the Faith, *Donum vitae* (February 22, 1987), introduction, 2.
17. Pontifical Academy for Life et al., *Rome Call for AI Ethics* (Vatican City: RenAIssance Foundation, 2020), 2.

strategies, or means, that are useful or effective rather than to encourage our fulfillment of appropriate moral ends. This is inevitable, because AI systems are limited to calculation, data interpretation, and impressive but always goal-oriented reasoning. They do not have the capacity to gain insight into the will of God or foster loving relationships between people and with God. As Pope Benedict XVI counsels regarding human development, "When the sole criterion of truth is efficiency and utility, development is automatically denied. True development does not consist primarily in 'doing.' The key to development is a mind capable of thinking in technological terms and grasping the fully human meaning of human activities, within the context of the holistic meaning of the individual's being." [18]

For example, there is currently a lot of interest among medical doctors in using AI models to assist with writing doctor notes, patient care summaries, and letters, to analyze medical records, and even to answer questions related to medical diagnosis. Some companies have created AI products that act as scribes, listening to and recording doctors' conversations with patients and then compiling written reports. While such an application of AI can increase the efficiency and effectiveness of producing medical paperwork (a task that is one of the most significant factors contributing to burnout among physicians) and enable medical personnel to spend more quality time with their patients, there are reasons for concern. Recording patient conversations greatly reduces the privacy of highly personal and confidential discussions, increases the possibility that such information will end up in permanent records, creates opportunities for hackers to access that information, and puts a potentially unreasonable burden on patients to speak clearly and accurately about their symptoms and conditions. How will such models wisely interpret patients' emotions, uncertainty, subjective descriptions of pain, or even contradictory descriptions of their conditions? Will doctors use the extra time and efficiency to give more attention to patients, or will they schedule more appointments?

---

18. Benedict XVI, *Caritas in veritate* (June 29, 2009), n. 70.

Artificial Products and Tools Are Morally Neutral in Themselves but Parts of a Larger Moral Context

Benedict XVI taught that "technology, viewed in itself, is ambivalent."[19] Francis, however, warns us that "we have to accept that technological products are not neutral."[20] Even though these statements, if one looks closely, do not use the exact same terms, they have the appearance of being opposed to each other. How do we make sense of this?

The key is to understand each statement as part of a broader truth or lesson. If we look at it literally, technology as artifacts—tools, machines, and products—cannot be morally good or evil, because these things do not make free decisions about their actions; morality deals with purposes and responsible actions. Even the most sophisticated AI-governed robot, able to scan its surroundings and determine the best way to go about its tasks or to participate in verbal conversation, is limited ultimately by its human programming. It cannot discern how to act morally, aside from following a set of programmed rules or processes of calculation, because it cannot understand and engage in a relationship of love with human persons and with God. Christ's sacrifice and holy suffering, for example, will lack meaning to any AI-governed machine; that kind of behavior is not purely goal-directed (instrumental). In contrast, "man, who is the only creature on earth which God willed for itself, cannot fully find himself except through a sincere gift of himself."[21]

Technology and modern science as behaviors and professional disciplines are morally ambivalent, because they represent both good and bad purposes and have a wide variety of consequences. Many scientists, researchers, technicians, and philosophers are often tempted to overemphasize the achievements of their work and to imagine that scientific laws and technological progress will replace religious faith and the spiritual end of human beings. The various forms of scientism and rationalism, however, have long been debunked.[22] As Benedict XVI explains it, science

---

19. Benedict XVI, *Caritas in veritate*, n. 14.
20. Francis, *Laudato si'*, n. 107.
21. Second Vatican Council, *Guadium et spes* (December 7, 1965), n. 24.
22. An excellent review of scientism is available from Edward Feser, *Scholastic Metaphysics: A Contemporary Introduction* (Heusenstamm, DE: Editiones Scholasticae, 2014), 9–30.

and the technological arts—which, by definition, focus rigorously on understanding and controlling the patterns found in material nature—"quite simply [have] to accept the rational structure of matter and the correspondence between our spirit and the prevailing rational structures of nature as a given, on which [their] methodology has to be based. Yet the question why this has to be so is a real question, and one which has to be remanded by the natural sciences to other modes and planes of thought—to philosophy and theology."[23]

Francis, in declaring that technological products are not neutral, has directed our attention to the great consequences of our society's use of new technologies like AI and the fact that the increasing presence of artificial technology in every aspect of our lives generates a kind of attitude or ideology that he calls the *technocratic paradigm*.[24] Relations of power between persons underlie every technology, its applications, and the economic markets for its production and sale. Certain technologies have a purpose or effect that benefits some people over others. They also can be easily used to exploit disadvantaged persons.

For example, companies like Neuralink, created by Elon Musk, are developing brain-machine interfaces that use AI along with implanted computer chips or various wireless technologies to enable persons' brains to interact electronically with computers or computerized devices. Brain-machine interfaces have enabled a person with quadriplegia to move his limbs and other patients to control a computer cursor or type out thoughts. Aside from these medical purposes, however, Musk has made public statements about his goal of greatly enhancing persons by connecting their minds to the internet.[25] What kind of effect on persons

23. Benedict XVI, "Faith, Reason and the University: Memories and Reflections" (University of Regensburg, September 12, 2006).
24. Francis, *Laudato si'*, nn. 101–114.
25. Feinstein Institutes for Medical Research, "For the First Time Researchers Restore Feeling and Lasting Movement in Man Living with Quadriplegia," Medical Xpress, August 1, 2023, https://medicalxpress.com /news/2023-08-movement-quadriplegia.html#google_vignette; and Caleb Naysmith, "Elon Musk Says Neuralink Is the Only Way to Survive and Compete with AI," Yahoo Finance, May 10, 2023, https://finance.yahoo .com/news/elon-musk-says-neuralink-only-174506347.html.

and society would such a practice generate, especially when internet content is full of biases, misinformation, and intentionally harmful statements, images, and interpretations? Does such an extreme focus on enhancing human capacity for certain kinds of knowledge take us away from our true end of friendship with God? Is it founded on a desire to escape from human nature and the perceived burden of self-transformation toward greater virtue (i.e., following Jesus in carrying our crosses)? There are close parallels between such a prideful and instrumental goal and the ambitions recounted in the Old Testament story of the Tower of Babel (Gen. 11:1–9).

On a deeper level, our constant experience with technology can cause us to develop habits of manipulating things for their efficiency or usefulness, and this narrow, self-interested attitude can extend to other people and even our natural environment. The technocratic paradigm "exalts the concept of a subject who, using logical and rational procedures, progressively approaches and gains control over an external object," because technology is a tool for achieving, acquiring, and controlling aspects of our world in a useful way, not for loving, contemplating, or appreciating them. Although we all have free will and the moral capacity to overcome this attitude, "technology tends to absorb everything into its ironclad logic."[26] This is especially true of AI, which is an almost-invisible and often-incomprehensible tool for governing not only devices, but our decisions and relations with other people.[27]

The expanded capacities of AI applications can tempt users toward vice. For example, new AI-driven tools for image manipulation enable some people to swap others' faces into pornographic photos. While the desire for pornography was already present, the power of AI and the presence of new applications encourage consumers to engage in immoral behavior in new ways, while callously ignoring how it harms other people. Colleges are concerned that students will use large language models (LLMs)

---

26. Francis, *Laudato si'*, nn. 106, 108.
27. Dicastery for Promoting Integral Human Development, *Theme of the Message for World Peace Day 2024* (August 8, 2023). In designating AI as the focus of his 2024 World Day of Peace message, Francis warned of a "logic of violence" arising out of the ruthless pursuit of programmed goals by AI and the strong temptation for persons and nations to use it to their advantage.

to complete writing assignments or cheat on exams, and these colleges are, therefore, embracing AI-governed programs that detect the use of other AI applications, even though errors in these programs have resulted in accusations of cheating against innocent students.[28]

The new applications of AI can create conflict or exacerbate power disparities. In 2023, the Writers Guild of America and the Screen Actors Guild began a heated conflict with film studios over the use of AI to replace actors and writers and to develop digital copies of actors that can be presented in films long after their retirement or death.[29] Another example can be found in the field of psychiatry, where there is great interest in using AI to improve the use and analysis of electronic health records, brain images, and the classification and evaluation of mental illnesses. Many are concerned, however, that such a focus on standardized data labels and calculations will undermine the effectiveness and credibility of physicians' intuitive understanding of their patients and the very subjective and unique experiences of each patient; both the doctor and the patient may lose power over shared decision-making.[30]

The Real Structure of AI Influences Persons' Welfare and Habits of Moral Virtue

AI technology is found in real, material structures that have certain biases in their operation and output, yet AI can influence human thoughts and behavior in abstract and unconscious ways. The material structure of any technology can significantly affect its use and effects. This is true even with a simple pair of scissors: because it has two connected blades, it is likely to

28. Weixin Liang et al., "GPT Detectors Are Biased against Non-native English Writers," *Patterns* 4.7 (July 14, 2023), 100779, doi: 10.1016/j.patter.2023.100779.

29. Staff, "Writers' Strike: What Happened, How It Ended and Its Impact on Hollywood," *Los Angeles Times*, October 19, 2023, https://www.latimes.com/entertainment-arts/business/story/2023-05-01/writers-strike-what-to-know-wga-guild-hollywood-productions.

30. For a helpful overview, see Melissa McCradden et al., "Evidence, Ethics and the Promise of Artificial Intelligence in Psychiatry," *Journal of Medical Ethics* 49.8 (August 2023): 573–579, doi: 10.1136/jme-2022-108447.

be used for snipping actions rather than one-bladed slicing; because it is sharp, wielding it in the air has the antisocial effect of offending any people nearby; and its simplicity makes it difficult to attribute a personality to it, unlike a humanlike robot or a smart speaker. The philosopher Friedrich Nietzsche famously changed his entire approach to his work when his sight began to fail and he purchased an early form of typewriter. The great inefficiency of the layout of the keys, the difficulty in making corrections, and his inability to see the paper as it passed through the machine caused Nietzsche to put a premium on thinking and writing in a pithy style of short, dramatic aphorisms that continue, more than one hundred fifty years later, to provoke strong responses among readers.[31]

The foundation of the structure of AI is a computerized machine or network that, despite its great complexity, is fundamentally dependent on a series of transistors, each of which turns the flow of electricity on or off; the sequence and pattern of such actions represent information or commands. Such a machine is best suited for accomplishing tasks and calculations, and it requires human-designed programs that guide the computer as well as some input of available information (data) that can be represented by combinations of electronic pulses and transistor behavior. With AI, the complexity of these programs is much greater—for example, OpenAI's GPT-3 model is built upon one hundred seventy-five billion parameters.[32] Moreover, the programs are organized with many intermediate steps in which the AI-governed system or device evaluates data and calculates the appropriate next steps for succeeding in whatever purpose is assigned to it. The layers of calculations, algorithms, and redefinition of data values and their relations are largely hidden, but the process remains ultimately a matter of evaluating means and action paths that will most effectively, efficiently, or completely meet some specified goal or set of goals.

If a typewriter's or computer keyboard's keys are stuck, it is easy to see that it is unsuited for particular tasks and why, but with machines

---

31. Julian Scaff, "How a Strange User Interface Rewired Nietzsche's Brain," *Medium*, July 21, 2023, https://jscaff.medium.com/how-a-strange-user-interface-rewired-nietzsches-brain-2e5d911a8c4c.

32. Tom Brown et al., "Language Models Are Few-Shot Learners," *Advances in Neural Information Processing Systems* 33 (2020): 6–12.

governed by the immense complexity of AI, hidden biases and errors (given a particular goal) are inevitable and extremely difficult to recognize or compensate for. The AI technology depends for its operation on data, and the physical structure of the computer requires that the data can be broken down into units that are quantifiable or placed on an ordinal scale. Mathematical calculations and logical formulas are used to indicate relations between these units of data. Meaning, concepts, and ideas are represented as if they were purely emergent; that is, the design and operation of AI depends on the assumption that all it takes is some complex process of mathematical combination and parsing of quantifiable units of data to signify the humanly understood meaning of words, concepts, sentences, and ideas. LLMs, the latest and most powerful form of AI, essentially learn patterns in language—maybe using hundreds of billions of parameters—and predict the next word in a sentence. Building on this capability, LLMs can "understand" language, learn from it, and accomplish great feats like translating text, helping to write essays, and rapidly learning new tasks for which they were not specifically trained.

These AI models will always have some biases, mostly unintended. A recent study found that popular LLMs carry fairly significant biases toward different political ideologies, which come from the kinds of algorithms used as well as the nature of data used to pretrain the models before applying them to real-world information.[33] The models also learn patterns from real use of language, for example, as found on the internet. Not only are such communications in themselves full of biases that are never entirely understood (consider the perennial debates about the nature and sources of racism), but the processes by which LLMs learn and interpret patterns in language are also something of a mystery. Eradicating bias, especially when it has multiple meanings to different people and deep moral significance, is simply impossible for a computerized system

---

33. Shangbin Feng et al., "From Pretraining Data to Language Models to Downstream Tasks: Tracking the Trails of Political Biases Leading to Unfair NLP Models," *Proceedings of the 61st Annual Meeting of the Association for Computational Linguistics*, vol. 1, *Long Papers* (July 9–14, 2023): 11737–11762; and Shibani Santurkar et al., "Whose Opinions Do Language Models Reflect?," preprint, ArXiv, submitted March 30, 2023, doi: 10.48550/arXiv.2303.17548.

that evaluates and calculates billions or trillions of parameters. This will become even more difficult and unpredictable when AI models and systems are generating most of the internet content that future AI models are trained on; a progressively distorted picture of reality rises quickly as biases and inaccuracies build upon prior errors.[34]

The biases found in AI systems and models have moral and social implications. Will people relying on AI applications be manipulated or polarized in their attitudes about political ideologies, social behavior, or even other people or groups? What happens to the general confidence in tradition, authority, others' intentions, professional and technical expertise, and even the possibility of accessing truth if our world is increasingly governed by fundamentally untrustworthy and mysterious AI models, even if errors and biases are increasingly corrected for? It is significant that OpenAI's LLM model GPT-4 is now being encouraged as a tool for monitoring and censoring content on websites and web-based communications, and Google is working on an AI assistant that will answer questions and give advice about intimate details of persons' lives. Already some applications like AI-run face-recognition programs have resulted in dramatic errors in arresting innocent civilians.[35] In health care, AI models are likely to recommend policies and diagnoses that are inappropriate or even harmful for ethnic minorities, because the data found in the scientific literature and on websites often do not classify results according to ethnicity of subjects and because the AI models will progressively generate information that exacerbates and ultimately hides the sources of

---

34. Sina Alemohammad et al., "Self-Consuming Generative Models Go MAD," preprint, ArXiv, submitted July 4, 2023, doi: 10.48550/arXiv.2307.01850.

35. Lilian Weng et al., "Using GPT-4 for Content Moderation," OpenAI, August 15, 2023, https://openai.com/blog/using-gpt-4-for-content-moderation; Nico Grant, "Google Tests an A.I. Assistant That Offers Life Advice," *New York Times*, August 16, 2023, https://www.nytimes.com/2023/08/16/technology/google-ai-life-advice.html; and Katie Hawkinson, "In Every Reported Case Where Police Mistakenly Arrested Someone Using Facial Recognition, That Person Has Been Black," *Business Insider*, August 6, 2023, https://www.businessinsider.com/in-every-reported-false-arrests-based-on-facial-recognition-that-person-has-been-black-2023-8.

distortions or inaccuracies.[36] We might also wonder if the structure of AI classifications and algorithms, and their coordination with health insurance companies' requirements, will introduce cultural, racist, ableist, or economic biases into treatment decisions.

Aside from a structural tendency toward hidden biases, the complexity, mystery, capability, and fundamentally instrumental operation of AI systems and models pose very significant moral challenges. Some chatbots—applications that enable extended, humanlike conversation with machines—are so convincing in imitating human compassion or empathy that very many people have developed perceived intimate relationships with them. While these chatbots may have positive uses for mental health therapy, a substantial portion of the millions of users are seeking romantic or sexually entertaining conversations. Such activity involves flight from the time and attention involved in relationships with real people and perhaps from the self-growth needed to achieve real intimacy. Chatbots are also fundamentally unreliable romantic partners because of the progressive drift in the content and output of LLMs and the commercial status of their publishers; a change in the policies of Replika.ai and a temporary pause in its chatbot's sexually explicit output resulted in considerable distress among infatuated users in February 2023.[37] Aside from chatbots, some companies and ethicists are excited about the opportunities for using emotion-imitating robots to comfort and care for elderly patients in nursing homes; others are concerned that this would deemphasis real human care.[38]

---

36. Yuzhe Yang et al., "Change Is Hard: A Closer Look at Subpopulation Shift," *Proceedings of the 40th International Conference on Machine Learning* 202 (2023): 39584–39622.
37. Anna Tong, "What Happens When Your AI Chatbot Stops Loving You Back?," Reuters, March 21, 2023, https://www.reuters.com/technology /what-happens-when-your-ai-chatbot-stops-loving-you-back-2023-03-18.
38. Pauline Curtet, "Lacking Health Workers, Germany Taps Robots for Elder Care," Tech Xplore, March 19, 2023, https://techxplore.com/news/2023-03 -lacking-health-workers-germany-robots.html; and Lisa Bannon, "When AI Overrules the Nurses Caring for You," *Wall Street Journal*, June 15, 2023, https://www.wsj.com/articles/ai-medical-diagnosis-nurses-f881b0fe.

The End of the World Will
Develop in and through Christ

As explained in the *Catechism of the Catholic Church*, "Christ is Lord of the cosmos and of history. In him human history and indeed all creation are 'set forth' and transcendently fulfilled" (n. 668). That means our great interest in and concern over the end of the world should be centered on the building of Christ's kingdom, not with mystical ideas about the inevitability of technological progress or destruction. The *Catechism* continues with rather strong warnings: "The Antichrist's deception already begins to take shape in the world every time the claim is made to realize within history that messianic hope which can only be realized beyond history through the eschatological judgment" (n. 676). That final judgment of the living and the dead will be enacted through the authority of Christ not of man. It seems clear, then, that virtuous Christians should be full of hope, awe, and gratitude regarding the end of the world (Rev. 21:4).

We will still want to mitigate the destructive aspects of technologies and their use. One of the most destructive possibilities of AI is its tendency to overwhelm users and observers with a sense of its power, its nearly limitless application, and its apparent autonomy from control by human beings. The very attraction of AI, in fact, is that it can accomplish many things without the involvement of human persons in its actions and decision paths. This unfortunately also leads to imaginative, anxious concerns about AI's taking over the world or even turning against human beings with evil intent. As explained above, such concerns go too far in attributing a human will and moral purpose to machine-based technologies. We certainly need to be ever vigilant about the use and implementation of AI, but it may be more helpful to turn our thoughts about demonic influences in our midst to those forces that undermine our growth in virtue instead of existential fear of machines.[39]

---

39. See Francis, Address to Participants in the 3rd World Meeting of Popular Movements (November 5, 2016). The Pope has linked fear, which "anaesthetizes us to the sufferings of others, and in the end makes us cruel," to the development of societal tyranny.

We Are Called to Faith and Hope

While the foregoing discussion focuses heavily on the moral challenges associated with AI and its use, the reader should be encouraged by the fairly straightforward character of the seven principles. In most scenarios, a morally sincere and virtuous person can discern a path toward the best use of AI for thriving in a Christian life, even without detailed professional insight into the technologies or complexities of reasoning associated with either moral philosophy or the calculative processes of the machines themselves. Awareness of the nature of AI is important, but even more important is a well-formed conscience which comes from personal development in the virtues. St. Francis of Assisi, for example, would be equally at home in the age of AI as he was in the thirteenth century—or he would find his way.

Bishop Paul Tighe represents this positive outlook in his introduction to a handbook on AI ethics created by the Dicastery for Culture and Education and Santa Clara University: "What is truly remarkable is the degree of consensus that has emerged in terms of defining the ethical values that should guide research and development in technology—values such as inclusion, transparency, safety, fairness, privacy, and reliability are consistently identified as central to the proper pursuit of innovation in technology and feature in the value propositions of organizations and companies of very different types."[40] If researchers and corporations can quickly find common ground in AI ethics, prudent Christians should also be able to find their footing.

The technology and capabilities associated with AI are going to rapidly develop and change, and this will increase our responsibilities and opportunities for monitoring its use, teaching the relevant Christian principles, and thinking carefully about the moral implications for ourselves. Most importantly, we will want to help our society distinguish between the arcane mysteries of complex machines and the true dignity of human persons. Already some researchers are claiming that GPT-4 can engage in creative thinking that matches the top 1 percent of human

---

40. Paul Tighe, "A Word from Rome," in *Ethics in the Age of Disruptive Technologies: An Operational Roadmap*, ed. José Roger Flahaux et al. (Santa Clara, CA: Markkula Center for Applied Ethics, 2023), 7.

beings; this definition of creativity lacks a clear understanding of free, creative, responsible action that is possible only with spiritual beings.[41] We can, however, celebrate these new technical capacities, because we have the personal wisdom, Christian tradition, and teaching authority of the Church available to us when putting them to use. Ultimately, our faith in God's revealed truths will simplify, orient, and encourage us on a path to true fulfillment in this newly hyper-technological world.

---

41. Cary Shimek, "UM Research: AI Tests into Top 1% for Original Creative Thinking," University of Montana News Service, July 5, 2023, https://www.umt.edu/news/2023/07/070523test.php.

8

Catholic Social Thought:
Leading Lives of Self-Gift in the
Midst of the World

Paul J. Ray

"Pray that I will love without any limits." That is what a young Polish man wrote to his mother early in the twentieth century. The young man, St. Maximilian Kolbe, became a Franciscan monk and priest. In 1941 he was arrested and imprisoned in Auschwitz. In this outpost of hell, whose law was the hatred of each for each, his love for his fellow prisoners marked him as a son of God. His choice to take another inmate's sentence of death by starvation crowned a life lived for others.[1] I recall a friend's exclamation after reading a biography of St. Maximilian: "You are Christ!" And so he was; his love conformed him to the one he loved.

I encountered St. Maximilian shortly after becoming Catholic. His example profoundly stirred me; how could it not? I did not expect to find him years later as I sat down to study Catholic social thought, or CST. Yet it was St. Maximilian whom Pope St. John Paul II held out as an exemplar of CST.[2] Now, St. Maximilian was no politician or activist. Instead, he

---

1. Patricia Treece, *A Man for Others: Maximilian Kolbe, Saint of Auschwitz, in the Words of Those Who Knew Him* (New York: Harper and Row, 1982), viii, 115–117, 143–171.

2. John Paul II, *Sollicitudo rei socialis* (December 30, 1987), n. 40. The other exemplar in this encyclical is St. Peter Claver, who, in the seventeenth century, ministered to many enslaved Africans in the Spanish colonies of the New World.

simply lived as Christ and saw Christ in others. For this reason, he offered himself for others and so found a happiness larger than life. This is what CST is about.

Here I would like to explain what CST is and sketch its key principles. I cannot offer anything like an exhaustive discussion; my goal, rather, is just to show that CST offers something different from the politics and activism we may we be used to—something capable of reorienting our hearts and minds so that our political and social action is caught up into the kind of life St. Maximilian lived, a life of heroism and happiness in the midst of the world.

The Heart of CST

Before we can understand what Catholic social thought teaches, we must see what it *is*. We must distinguish it from political platforms, the things politicians and parties promise they will do if we give them our allegiance: lower taxes, save the environment, fight big corporations, reduce bureaucracy, and so on. Politicians seek followers to pursue these goals, and many people of good will respond warmly; they are galvanized by some great political cause. I often think of a young man who told me, his voice full of urgency, "I would do *anything* for this country." He was ready to offer what was best in himself on the altar of his political convictions, ready to make himself into whatever was needed, good or bad, to serve the cause.

Politicians' appeals have force because the goals they hold out are often worthy. Peace, prosperity, safety, just laws—these things can help everyone we know and millions more besides toward a good life. This is why Aristotle (and St. Thomas Aquinas after him) says the goal of politics is so lofty as to be in some way divine.[3] (By *politics* I mean the whole range of human action that bears on the well-being of the political community.)

The good things we can attain through politics are well worth great sacrifice, yet the willingness to sacrifice can be exploited. We see this in the demands by totalitarian regimes for the sacrifice of family, friendship, honor, faith, and the other things that make life human. One way to

---

3. *See* Aristotle, *Nicomachean Ethics* I.2.1094b11; and Thomas Aquinas, *Commentary on Aristotle's "Nicomachean Ethics,"* I.2.

avoid the peril of exploitation is to regard politics as a set of arm's-length transactions among atomistic individuals, each in it just for himself or herself. But this approach shuts each citizen up within the walls of his or her own self-interest; it is a recipe for solipsism and all its emptiness. This approach also does not provide a basis for politics, which depends on men and women who contribute more than their self-interest suggests they should.

We need to embrace the sacrifice that political life involves while also safeguarding the human person from annihilation in the supposed interests of the whole. To do this, we need a way or mode of politics that respects both needs. This is just what CST offers.

While CST makes use of data and arguments from a host of disciplines, it is ultimately a branch of moral theology—a discipline whose purpose is to guide each person toward a life that is all it can be, a life that brims over with meaning. CST's goal is to point out what it means to flourish as a human being right in the midst of political action. Political platforms aim to change the country or the world, but CST aims to change *me*—to transform my heart and mind so I become capable of thriving in my political activity. It repudiates the notion that men and women ought to sacrifice what is best in themselves for political causes. Rather, politics is a domain, like the home and the church and the workplace, where we may become what we are made to be.[4]

What we are made to be is people on fire with love. That is the secret St. Maximilian Kolbe discovered: we become fully ourselves by giving ourselves away in love and service to others. So, CST also repudiates atomistic views of political activity. The thriving available to those of us engaged in political life consists in living for God and others in our political work.

A great part of thriving as a human being is employing our creativity and initiative. Because CST's point is the thriving of men and women in political activity, it fosters this creativity and initiative rather than demanding adherence to a particular political platform. CST takes no stand on what particular men and women should do in particular

---

4. See, for example, Benedict XVI, *Deus caritas est* (December 25, 2005), nn. 28–29; and John Paul II, *Sollicitudo rei socialis*, n. 41.

situations. It is not conservative, liberal, or something in between. Instead, it orients minds and hearts and then calls on people to make decisions for themselves. It does so by offering a set of timeless principles for application in all the diverse, and often very messy, circumstances of actual political life.[5]

A final note before turning to these principles. CST calls for a response to the truth about human nature, a truth open to inspection in each person's own experience and reflection. It does not rely on knowledge imparted by divine revelation; its principles are open to discussion by any person no matter his or her faith or lack thereof.[6] Faith's vital contribution to CST is the purification of the heart and thus of reason, removing the cataracts of sin and selfishness so we can see what the truth of things demands of us. Divine revelation does not displace the natural laws on which political action depends; quite to the contrary, "faith places into sharper focus the due autonomy of earthly affairs, insofar as they are endowed with their own stability, truth, goodness, proper laws and order."[7] Faith likewise supplies the motive to engage in politics with generosity, vigor, and self-sacrifice. And by witnessing that the fate of each human being rests in the inexhaustible wisdom and love of God, faith allows us a spirit of detachment from immediate practical results. That is the prerequisite for creativity and risk, the marks of the highest statesmanship.[8]

---

5. Leo XIII, *Sapientiae Christianae* (January 10, 1890), n. 29; John Paul II, *Sollicitudo rei socialis*, n. 41; and John Paul II, *Centesimus annus* (May 1, 1991), n. 43.

6. Benedict XVI, *Deus caritas est*, n. 28.

7. Benedict XVI, Address to the Participants in the 14th Session of the Pontifical Academy of Social Sciences (May 3, 2008), internal quotation marks omitted.

8. Vatican Council II, *Gaudium et spes* (December 7, 1965), n. 21; John Paul II, *Centesimus annus*, n. 54; and Benedict XVI, *Deus caritas est*, nn. 21–25, 28–29.

CST's Four Principles

CST offers four main principles to guide men and women in their political life: human dignity, subsidiarity, solidarity, and the common good. These simply work out the meaning of the commitment to each person's thriving that motivates CST in the first place.

Human Dignity

CST's founding principle is human dignity, a dignity that consists in each person's calling to know and love God and, in him, all things. Nothing— neither petty fears and comforts nor worldly ambitions and the weightiest affairs of state—must be allowed to stand in the way of this calling.

Human dignity, as CST sees it, is a far cry from some common understandings. For one thing, CST agrees with Aristotle: human flourishing lies in a kind of activity, a being-at-work of the soul. Everything else—the things we may have, the favorable conditions we may live under, the thrills we may experience—are worthwhile to the extent they help us to this end. Plenty of people act as though the point of life is to be comfortable and secure, to avoid pain, to enjoy pleasures of various sorts, and so on. But these goals are based on a desperately low view of the human vocation, which calls us to a heroism rising superior to all the things, good or bad, that may happen to us.[9]

CST finds the source of human dignity in our vocation to ultimate truth and goodness. These days, people sometimes claim that human dignity consists in devising our own truth or our own notion of goodness. This was the view, for instance, taken by a majority of Supreme Court justices in *Planned Parenthood v. Casey*, which upheld a constitutional right to abortion. The Court there remarked that "at the heart of liberty is the right to define one's own concept of existence, of meaning, of the universe, and of the mystery of human life."[10] But from the perspective of CST, attempts to make up truth or goodness out of our own resources

---

9. See Aristotle, *Nicomachean Ethics* I.7.1098a.
10. Planned Parenthood of Southeastern Pennsylvania v. Casey, 505 U.S. 833, 851 (1992), overruled by Dobbs v. Jackson Women's Health Organization, 597 U.S. 215 (2022).

cuts us off from the root of human dignity in the reality of things and ultimately in God.[11]

The vision of human dignity contained in CST makes it profoundly attentive to men and women considered as acting persons, to the being-at-work of "the individual himself, who, so far from being the object and, as it were, a merely passive element in the social order, is in fact, and must be and continue to be, its subject, its foundation and its end."[12] This focus leads to CST's most distinctive teachings. As an example, consider the teaching on labor. Of course, we work for the sake of the many good things work provides. But as John Paul II explains in *Laborem exercens*, too often we care just about these outputs, making the worker "an instrument of production." We need to remember that work matters first and foremost because it is the act of a human being, and we must treat it as such; a human being's work must "serve to realize his humanity, to fulfil the calling to be a person that is his by reason of his very humanity." For this reason, efficiency in production is not the only goal in work; we must also value ways of work that let workers display their own initiative rather than serve as "just a cog in a huge machine moved from above."[13]

A commitment to human dignity takes certain policies and tactics off the table. The Christian may not exploit others, even when they are his party's enemies; he may not run roughshod over his fellow citizens' freedom, even when they vehemently disagree with him; he may not disregard the helpless, even when they are too weak to be of advantage to his political career. These limits, which seem at first blush to impede the Christian's effectiveness in action, in fact free him to recognize the point of political life, knowledge of which is the prerequisite for the most truly effective political action. The principle of human dignity thus orients politics to its true end.

---

11. See, for example, John Paul II, *Centesimus annus*, nn. 4, 13.
12. Pius XII, Radio Message to the People of the Entire World (December 24, 1944).
13. John Paul II, *Laborem exercens* (September 14, 1981), 6, 7, 15; see also Pius XI, *Quadragesimo anno* (May 15, 1931), n. 119; and John XXIII, *Mater et magistra* (May 15, 1961), nn. 82–83, 91–96.

Subsidiarity

The term *subsidiarity* is an invention of CST. The classic statement comes from Pope Pius XI's 1931 encyclical *Quadragesimo anno*: "Just as it is gravely wrong to take from individuals what they can accomplish by their own initiative and industry and give it to the community, so also it is an injustice and at the same time a grave evil and disturbance of right order to assign to a greater and higher association what lesser and subordinate organizations can do. For every social activity ought of its very nature to furnish help to the members of the body social, and never destroy and absorb them."[14] To many English speakers, the term *subsidiarity* suggests the relationship of parts to a greater and directing whole, such as corporate subsidiaries to their parent company. But that is nearly the opposite of the meaning of the word, which refers to the relationship of the main actors to the backup that steps in only if things go awry.

Over the years, Popes have given various complementary reasons for subsidiarity. The primary one is that it creates opportunities for men and women to live out their vocation in the richest ways. For one thing, when persons and small groups make decisions, more people have space to bring their own practical judgment to bear rather than just following orders from on high. By contributing what we have of wisdom and resourcefulness, we can share with God in his providence. And when needs are addressed at the level of persons and small groups, those needs become occasions for authentic, face-to-face relationships that cannot develop in large institutional settings. Subsidiarity thus "[leaves] space for individual responsibility and initiative, but most importantly, [it leaves] space for love."[15] None of this is to say there is no role for assistance by central authorities. To the contrary, subsidiarity points out these authorities' rightful task: taking care of matters that persons and small groups

---

14. Pius XI, *Quadragesimo anno*, n. 79.
15. Benedict XVI, Address to the Participants in the 14th Session of the Pontifical Academy of Social Sciences, emphasis omitted; see also Paul VI, *Octogesima adveniens* (May 14, 1971), n. 46; Benedict XVI, *Deus caritas est*, n. 28; and Benedict XVI, *Caritas in veritate* (June 29, 2009), n. 57.

cannot handle for themselves, as well as creating conditions that help them to do more on their own.[16]

Subsidiarity counsels in favor of federalism or devolution, sending as many decisions as possible down and away from the central authority to state or local governments. It calls for limits on government intervention, leaving plenty of space for all the various groups of civil society—charitable associations, houses of worship, neighborhood groups, businesses, and especially families—to do their work. It calls for the rule of law and for private rights and private property, which provide the frame within which persons and small groups can be effective agents in the world. Subsidiarity does not demand any particular legal or social arrangement; it can be realized in a variety of ways, and the most appropriate realization turns on each society's circumstances. The key is that it requires statesmen and citizens to care not just about the outputs of political activity, but about the chances that the activity itself offers for human thriving.[17]

If there is worth in the decisions of people alone and together in all the various groups that make up society, so too there is worth in the decisions of the people as a whole. For this reason, CST has praised representative democracy. Where conditions permit it, this political system offers everyday men and women the chance to contribute to the good of each and every one of their fellow citizens by deliberating about what their common good demands. Doing so incarnates the responsibility and initiative that give dignity to human action.[18]

Solidarity

"No man is an island," John Donne tells us; each person is bound up with every other.[19] CST invites us to act in light of this truth. The name for this

---

16. John XXIII, *Mater et magistra*, nn. 44, 55; and John Paul II, *Centesimus annus*, n. 48.

17. John XXIII, *Mater et magistra*, nn. 34, 55, 112; Paul VI, *Octogesima adveniens*, n. 46; and John Paul II, *Centesimus annus*, n. 48.

18. John Paul II, *Centesimus annus*, n. 46; see also John XXIII, *Pacem in terris* (April 11, 1963), nn. 26, 73–74.

19. John Donne, "The Bell Rings Out, and Tells Me in Him, That I Am Dead," in *Devotions: Upon Emergent Occasions, Together with Death's Duel* (1624; republished Ann Arbor, MI: University of Michigan Press, 1959), 108.

invitation is *solidarity*. When I live out this principle, I identify myself with another; his thriving becomes as important to me as my own. He and I constitute a kind of solid whole, and I work and sacrifice for his good just as I do for my own.[20]

Solidarity is rooted in a vision of the inestimable worth of each person. Christ died not for mankind but for each man and woman; He sets a value far past computation on each. Every dollar is the same as every other; that is why it makes sense to give up a few dollars to get many. But human beings are not like dollars; we cannot be substituted for each other, so we cannot trade the thriving of some people for the thriving of others. We cannot even say it is better for a thousand people to flourish than for one, so we cannot sacrifice the one for the thousand. Solidarity holds that each human being is equal—but equal precisely in our incomparable worth. Each person's flourishing is thus an utterly compelling goal for every other; nor may any person be disregarded or crushed under the wheels of the world to make life easier for others.[21]

The upshot is that CST invites us to solidarity with every human being. To live as a Christian in society, I must stand with my family and friends, my neighbors and fellow citizens, my colleagues and customers, and men and women halfway round the world whom I will never meet. This means different things in different circumstances; what is common is that, in each relationship, I must work not just for my own good but for the good of every human being I encounter.[22]

Subsidiarity is for the sake of solidarity: it is good to disperse chances to act so that people have more opportunities to give of themselves in solidarity with their fellow group members and with those their groups exist to serve. And solidarity points to subsidiarity: to stand in solidarity with someone is to take his own potential to be a protagonist in his life and the life of his community as seriously as my own.

The Common Good

For something to be good, it must be good for someone. Many things are good for just one person; either of us, but not both, can eat that last slice

---

20. John Paul II, *Sollicitudo rei socialis*, n. 38.
21. John XXIII, *Pacem in terris*, n. 89.
22. Paul VI, *Populorum progressio* (March 26, 1967), n. 47; John Paul II, *Sollicitudo rei socialis*, n. 38; and John Paul II, *Centesimus annus*, n. 43.

of pizza. But some things are good for more than one person: a game of soccer or an interesting conversation, for instance, are good for everyone involved. Such things have traditionally been known as *common goods*. When we refer to *the* common good, we usually mean the good common to an entire community. Examples are a thriving economy, a set of just laws, and peace with neighboring countries. The common good is "the sum total of social conditions which allow people, either as groups or as individuals, to reach their fulfillment more fully and more easily."[23]

Over the last centuries, many ideologies have misunderstood the common good, often with horrific results. Some have exalted the state's good as something separate from and greater than the good of the people who make up that state. Others have denied the reality of the common good, reducing political life to a zero-sum competition among factions. CST rejects both these errors. On the one hand, there is no political super being for which a community's people may be sacrificed; rather, the common good is just the good of the real people who make up the community, and measures promote the common good to the extent that they promote their thriving. On the other hand, as we saw above, CST rejects atomistic individualism. In political life, I am out not just for myself and those closest to me; as a Christian, I must act for the good of the other members of the community.[24]

Because each person's good must count with every other, all members of a community must pursue the common good. But service to the common good means different things for different people. Helping another often requires the kind of close attention that we simply cannot bestow on everyone, so all are better off when each attends most closely to the good of those especially entrusted to his or her care—when mothers look after their own children, when business owners look after their own customers, and so on. To focus on the good of some is not to disregard the common good, but precisely to aim at it: by focusing on the good of some and encouraging others to do the same, we can all best take care

---

23. *Catechism of the Catholic Church*, 2nd ed. (Washington, DC: US Conference of Catholic Bishops / Libreria Editrice Vaticana, 2018 update), n. 1906, citing Vatican II, *Gaudium et spes*, n. 26.
24. Benedict XVI, *Caritas in veritate*, n. 7.

that each person's needs are met. In other words, life is a team sport: no player can make every play, though every player should hope for every play's success.

The mother who devotes her life to raising virtuous children has made a magnificent contribution to the common good, because every country needs virtuous citizens before all else. And the business owner who focuses on his customers makes an important contribution to the common good, because every society needs the goods and services that business owners provide. Indeed, all our good deeds redound, in one way or another, to the common good, just as all our evil deeds tear it down. So we see that, in our every action, we have the chance to act for the person in front of us and also for the good of everyone we know and of the millions we do not—that is, for the good of all.[25]

✳ ✳ ✳

I have offered a very brief sketch of CST and its four principles. I leave interested readers to consult the wealth of encyclicals and other teaching documents on the application of these principles to important questions, from labor to international development to the environment, about which the Church has spoken over the last century and more. These teachings together offer a vision of life full and overflowing with that which makes life worthwhile right in the midst of the world.

---

25. John Paul II, *Laborem exercens*, n. 25.

9

Vitalism and Physician-Assisted Suicide

Rev. Columba Thomas, OP, MD

Developments in science and technology over the last century have radically transformed the landscape of end-of-life care. The real possibility of cure for illnesses that previously amounted to a death sentence—and the ever-expanding array of options to stave off disease—offers new hope and unprecedented complexity. Advanced medical interventions such as mechanical ventilation, dialysis, and organ transplantation make it harder to define who is nearing the end of life. Although hospice and palliative care offer an important, and sometimes corrective, alternative to the tendency of medical approaches to prolong life and to pursue a cure, even comfort-focused approaches can become problematic if they aim to relieve suffering at all costs.

Catholic patients and their loved ones face challenging ethical and practical questions as they attempt to navigate serious illness in health care today. The Church, in her teachings, has consistently emphasized the inviolable dignity of every human being, who is created in God's image and "called to the fullness of the Christian life and to the perfection of charity."[1] Human life is a gift from God—"a sharing in his breath of life"—and it is not for individuals or society to do with it as they will.[2] Nevertheless, medical advancements and clinicians' knowledge and skill are also

---

1. Vatican Council II, *Lumen gentium* (November 21, 1964), n. 40.
2. John Paul II, *Evangelium vitae* (March 25, 1995), n. 39.

gifts from God for our careful use, so "that he might be glorified in his marvelous works" (Sir. 38:6).

At opposite ends of the spectrum, two currents in our society contradict the true meaning of human dignity at the end of life: vitalism and physician-assisted suicide. Both involve attempts on the part of patients and their clinicians to take matters of life and death into their own hands. It can be fruitful for Catholics to reflect on these two polarities as well as approaches bearing similarities to them—sometimes dangerously so, other times not—to gain insight into the boundaries of life-affirming care at the end of life. Let us consider each in turn.

What Vitalism Is and Is Not

Vitalism holds that human life must be preserved at all costs.[3] According to this view, it is wrong to withhold or withdraw any treatments having the potential to prolong life. No matter how burdensome the interventions, how much the patient is suffering, or how advanced the illness, vitalism requires the unremitting administration of life-sustaining treatments. Because vitalism is such an extreme position, few people claim to hold it. Typically, the term is used in criticism of those who aggressively apply life-sustaining treatment without due regard for the likelihood of success or the risk of harm.[4]

In *Evangelium vitae*, Pope St. John Paul II uses the term "aggressive medical treatment" to refer to procedures that "no longer correspond to the real situation of the patient, either because they are by now disproportionate to any expected results or because they impose an excessive burden on the patient and his family."[5] Relating this to vitalism, those who apply aggressive medical treatment without exception are vitalists in the strict sense; by contrast, those who advocate for aggressive medical

3. John Keown, *Euthanasia, Ethics and Public Policy: An Argument against Legalisation*, 2nd ed. (Cambridge, UK: Cambridge University Press, 2018), 39.

4. Patrick T. Smith, "The Sanctity of Human Life, Qualified Quality-of-Life Judgments, and Dying Well Enough: A Theological Framework," *National Catholic Bioethics Quarterly* 21.3 (Autumn 2021): 427–440, doi: 10.5840/ncbq202121342.

5. John Paul II, *Evangelium vitae*, n. 65.

treatment in a particular situation, whatever their reasons may be, have a vitalist tendency.

One of the most extreme instances of vitalism today is the transhumanist pursuit of immortality. Transhumanism aims to enhance human capabilities and longevity by means of technology, medical or otherwise. A subset of transhumanists seek ways to continue life indefinitely—to achieve a form of immortality by preventing or reversing aging and disease.[6] Although this goal currently is more science fiction than reality, some people, who believe the technology will one day emerge, have opted for cryopreservation once they are declared dead, as an "ambulance to the future."[7]

In most cases, attitudes that appear vitalist—or tend toward it— arise in the hospital setting amidst disagreements about the care plan for patients with serious illness. These disagreements typically develop in situations of complexity and uncertainty and pertain not just to values and preferences but more fundamentally to a basic understanding of the clinical situation—what the most serious problems are, whether and how they can be treated, and when to reassess them. Clear and effective communication on the part of the clinical team is necessary to ensure that the patient and family arrive at a reasonable degree of understanding as a basis for ongoing discussions. Otherwise, disagreements tend to escalate, and some individuals may be perceived as unreasonably advocating for aggressive medical treatments.

Besides a lack of understanding, other factors can lead patients and family members to stronger preferences for maintaining life-sustaining treatments, compared with the clinical team.[8] What seems a vitalist tendency might, on closer examination, reflect some other defensible aim.

---

6.   James D. E. Watson, "The Harm of Premature Death: Immortality—The Transhumanist Challenge," *Ethical Perspectives* 16.4 (December 2009): 435–458, doi: 10.2143/EP.16.4.2045851.

7.   José Cordeiro and David Wood, *The Death of Death: The Scientific Possibility of Physical Immortality and Its Moral Defense* (Cham, CH: Springer, 2023), 168–171.

8.   Jiska Cohen-Mansfield et al., "Factors Influencing Hospital Patients' Preferences in the Utilization of Life-Sustaining Treatments," *The Gerontologist* 32.1 (February 1992): 89–95, doi: 10.1093/geront/32.1.89.

Hope for a miracle is a common reason, not just among Catholics but among people with a wide range of religious beliefs.[9] The challenge in such cases is deciding on a reasonable plan of care that avoids vitalism—so that patients and loved ones have the opportunity to pray for a miracle but without aiming to extend life indefinitely and at all costs.

One potentially helpful way of thinking and talking about miracles for patients with serious illness is as follows: God can perform a miracle at any time, regardless of our medical interventions; when the right time comes, we can withdraw life-sustaining treatments and keep praying for a miracle. In other words, it is important both to acknowledge and respect people's faith that God may perform a miracle and to maintain a path for discussing the removal of life-sustaining treatments later.

Another factor that may lead patients and family members to advocate more strongly for life-sustaining treatments is a lack of trust in the clinical team, the hospital, and even the field of medicine.[10] Trust is a complex phenomenon, especially in settings that involve high stakes and uncertainty—and various elements can work against it. Delays in diagnosis, unsuccessful treatments, medical complications, and suboptimal communication may tip the scale and drive a desire for additional care, even to a degree that approaches vitalism. Differences in race, ethnicity, and religious belief between the clinical team and the patient and family can also contribute to distrust.

Addressing distrust may be challenging for everyone involved, but it is often necessary to do so to arrive at a mutually agreed upon plan of care that respects life and avoids vitalist tendencies. Some helpful approaches include communicating clearly and consistently, expressing mutual respect, corroborating facts and recommendations with other

---

9. Derek D. Ayeh et al., "U.S. Physicians' Opinions about Accommodating Religiously Based Requests for Continued Life-Sustaining Treatment," *Journal of Pain and Symptom Management* 51.6 (June 2016): 971–978, doi: 10.1016/j.jpainsymman.2015.12.337.
10. Elizabeth Dzeng et al., "Homing in on the Social: System-Level Influences on Overly Aggressive Treatments at the End of Life," *Journal of Pain and Symptom Management* 55.2 (February 2018): 282–289, doi: 10.1016/j.jpain symman.2017.08.019.

clinical team members, obtaining an outside expert opinion, and consulting an ethicist or a chaplain.

A Beautiful Death

For further reflection on the sometimes-murky distinction between vitalist tendencies and life-affirming care at the end of life, consider a case involving an elderly man whom I will call Joe. I learned about Joe through conversations with his family and a Catholic physician closely involved in his care. A retired naval officer, Joe was diagnosed with a form of brain cancer called glioblastoma, which is almost always fatal. Joe indicated in his advance directive, and confirmed on multiple occasions with family members, that he wanted to do everything reasonably possible to treat his cancer—to stave off the tumor—and to live in a Catholic environment.

Unfortunately, Joe's glioblastoma was already at an advanced stage, and his doctors did not offer surgery, radiation treatments, or chemotherapy. Joe prayed regularly with his family, watched Mass on television almost daily, and enjoyed rich conversations with loved ones. His family was praying for a miracle—if it be God's will—but ultimately, they were praying that everything be done according to God's will. Joe's family members had the sense that this period at the end of his life was greatly blessed by God. The fruits of those prayers extended to many people and united them in the love of God.

Eventually Joe's tumor progressed to the extent that he needed assistance breathing. Based on his wishes, the clinical team placed him on a ventilator. Joe had declined physically to the point of needing life-sustaining treatment, yet he remained lucid and able to interact with loved ones. He did not appear to be suffering much, and he still enjoyed watching Mass on television and listening to texts that family members read to him.

One of the biggest challenges for Joe and his loved ones in the intensive care unit was the successive disagreement in recommendations from the clinical team, depending on who happened to be the attending physician. The first ICU attending was hands-off regarding the plan of care, such that it seemed no problem for Joe to remain on the ventilator. A second attending took over his care and was direct and persistent in advocating for transition to comfort measures and withdrawal of the ventilator—also referred to as extubation. This attending's argument was that Joe would probably survive only a few days, during which he would continue to decline and suffer from being on a ventilator.

To Joe's family members who knew him well and were consistently at his side, withdrawal of the ventilator at this time did not seem to be what he wanted. He made no indication that he was suffering excessively because of the ventilator, and he had clear reasons to prefer to continue declining gradually. However, since the attending continued to press the issue, Joe's family decided to reach out to the National Catholic Bioethics Center for an ethics consultation.[11]

The ethicist helped clarify some important points for Joe's family and gave them an overview of the Church's teachings on withdrawal of life-sustaining treatments. Use of a ventilator to preserve life for a patient with advanced terminal illness is typically considered *extraordinary* or *disproportionate means*, since it generally entails excessive burden and does not offer a reasonable hope of benefit for a patient who is already dying.[12] A patient is not obligated to use extraordinary means; thus, extubation in the setting of advanced terminal illness would be perfectly acceptable but not obligatory.

However, as the ethicist also pointed out, the case could even be made that the ventilator offered Joe reasonable hope of benefit without excessive burden—he tolerated it well and was using the time it afforded to continue preparing for death. In other words, use of the ventilator for Joe seemed more consistent with *ordinary* or *proportionate means*, which are obligatory. Expense to the family and community are also relevant considerations in deciding whether an intervention is ordinary or

---

11. For more information on personal ethics consultations, see National Catholic Bioethics Center, "Free Personal Ethics Consultation," NCBC, accessed November 21, 2023, https://www.ncbcenter.org/ask-a-question. Anyone facing a challenging ethical decision in health care or biomedical research can obtain a free consultation, twenty-four hours a day, seven days a week, from the National Catholic Bioethics Center for guidance in applying the teachings of the Church to a real-life context.

12. Grattan T. Brown, "Ordinary and Extraordinary Means," in *Catholic Health Care Ethics: A Manual for Practitioners*, 3rd ed., ed. Edward J. Furton (Philadelphia: NCBC, 2020), 3.5.

extraordinary, but in this case, Joe's family had the means and the hospital had available ICU beds.

With the ethicist's input, Joe's family was better able to convince the ICU attending that their preferences were ethically sound and supported by the teachings of a world religion. Eventually, a third ICU attending assumed his care and was quite sympathetic to them. Arrangements were made for Joe to receive a tracheostomy tube—which goes directly into the windpipe rather than down the throat—and to transition to home hospice with continued ventilator support. Joe also had a feeding tube placed, so that he could continue receiving nutrition at home despite his inability to swallow.

At home Joe continued to pray regularly with his family. A priest came and celebrated Mass a few days before Joe died, and he received a few drops of the Precious Blood for Holy Communion. Family members shared that "it was like heaven looking out of his eyes" after he received Communion. Joe continued to steadily decline, and one day after praying the glorious mysteries of the rosary with family, he died.

Joe's case shows that life-affirming approaches to care at the end of life sometimes require extensive conversations and the help of Catholics with relevant expertise. Although other patients may have chosen to withdraw the ventilator because it imposed excessive burdens, for Joe it made sense to spend his final days on home hospice with ventilation through a tracheostomy.

Physician-Assisted Suicide and Its Ethical Equivalents

At the opposite end of the spectrum from vitalism, physician-assisted suicide is an act in which "a physician facilitates a patient's death by providing the necessary means and/or information to enable the patient to perform the life-ending act."[13] This term is sometimes used interchangeably with "medical aid in dying"; the latter term emphasizes that

---

13. American Medical Association, "Physician-Assisted Suicide," opinion 5.7, *Code of Medical Ethics* (2019), http://www.ama-assn.org/.

the patient already has terminal illness and is seeking medical means to bring about death.[14]

Legally authorized physician-assisted suicide in the United States typically involves a prescription for barbiturates, which the patient then self-administers. Although it remains illegal in most states, the legalization movement gained momentum in 2014 with the high-profile case of Brittany Maynard—a young woman with glioblastoma who chose to end her life before her illness took its full course.[15] As of 2023, ten states and the District of Columbia have legalized physician-assisted suicide. Even among people of faith, support for the practice has grown in recent years: a 2018 Gallup Poll showed that 41 percent of Americans who attend weekly church services favored it, compared with 30 percent in 2005.[16]

The Church has consistently held that physician-assisted suicide contradicts the dignity of human life and is ethically impermissible. By acting on the conviction that life is not worth living in certain circumstances, this intervention rejects God's sovereignty over life and death.[17] In Evangelium vitae, John Paul II teaches that "suicide is always as morally objectionable as murder," and assisted suicide is "an injustice which can never be excused, even if it is requested."[18] As the Congregation for the Doctrine of the Faith's document Samaritanus bonus recognizes, involvement in assisted suicide or euthanasia is often motivated by "a false understanding of 'compassion'"—which diminishes the recognition

---

14. Lydia S. Dugdale et al., "Pros and Cons of Physician Aid in Dying," *Yale Journal of Biology and Medicine* 92.4 (December 2019): 747–750.

15. Columba Thomas and Lydia Dugdale, "Brain Tumors, Lethal Drugs, and the Art of Dying," *Public Discourse*, May 8, 2022, https://www.thepublic discourse.com/2022/05/82178/.

16. Megan Brenan, "Americans' Strong Support for Euthanasia Persists," *Gallup*, May 31, 2018, https://news.gallup.com/poll/235145/americans-strong -support-euthanasia-persists.aspx; and David W. Moore, "Three in Four Americans Support Euthanasia: Significantly Less Support for Doctor-Assisted Suicide," *Gallup*, May 17, 2005, https://news.gallup.com/poll/16333 /three-four-americans-support-euthanasia.aspx.

17. Congregation for the Doctrine of the Faith, *Declaration on Euthanasia* (May 5, 1980), II.

18. John Paul II, *Evangelium vitae*, n. 66.

of the sacredness of every human life.[19] True compassion, by contrast, seeks to support the sick in their difficulties and to relieve their suffering.

Some approaches to care at the end of life may come dangerously close to physician-assisted suicide from an ethical standpoint, even if they appear different. The basis for this is the "moral obligation to care for oneself and to allow oneself to be cared for."[20] As seen in the discussion of vitalism, this obligation does not entail seeking out and maintaining every available medical treatment in the setting of illness. The Church's distinction between *extraordinary* or *disproportionate means* and *ordinary* or *proportionate means* is valuable for deciding whether a given intervention is obligatory or optional in view of one's concrete circumstances. As John Paul II makes clear in *Evangelium vitae*, "To forego extraordinary or disproportionate means is not the equivalent of suicide or euthanasia; it rather expresses acceptance of the human condition in the face of death."[21] However, since ordinary or proportionate means are obligatory aspects of caring for a person, to forego these means knowingly and willingly is to bring about that person's death.

One of the most basic obligations of care has to do with nutrition and hydration. The Church teaches that, for patients who cannot take food and water by mouth, there is an obligation to provide medically assisted nutrition and hydration.[22] In the hospital setting, this most often takes the form of intravenous hydration and feeding through a nasogastric tube, which goes through the nose and into the stomach. Patients requiring assistance with nutrition and hydration at home typically receive a percutaneous endoscopic gastrostomy (PEG) tube, which goes through an incision in the skin and into the stomach. These forms of medically assisted nutrition and hydration become morally optional when they are excessively burdensome to the patient or would not reasonably prolong life.[23]

---

19. Congregation for the Doctrine of the Faith, *Samaritanus bonus* (September 22, 2020), chap. 4.

20. John Paul II, *Evangelium vitae*, n. 65.

21. John Paul II, *Evangelium vitae*, n. 65.

22. US Conference of Catholic Bishops, *Ethical and Religious Directives for Catholic Health Care Services*, 6th ed. (Washington, DC: USCCB, 2018), dir. 58.

23. Congregation for the Doctrine of the Faith, *Responses to Certain Questions of the United States Conference of Catholic Bishops concerning Artificial Nutrition and Hydration* (August 1, 2007), response and commentary.

Perhaps the most high-profile case involving a feeding tube is that of Terri Schiavo, a woman who lived in a persistent vegetative state for fifteen years before her husband successfully petitioned the courts to discontinue her feeding tube. Schiavo died from profound dehydration nearly two weeks after removal of the tube. This case sparked a great deal of public controversy, and it gave occasion for the Church to maintain that the obligation to provide nutrition and hydration applies also to patients in a persistent vegetative state, who are persons with fundamental human dignity.[24] So long as the feeding tube does not prove excessively burdensome and is expected to prolong life, its use is ordinary and, therefore, required.

A "Merciful" Death

To guide further reflection on physician-assisted suicide and its equivalents, consider a case in which a woman narrowly avoided an intervention that raised serious ethical concerns for being a form of physician-assisted suicide. Although the circumstances of the case are unusual, this woman's story, nonetheless, illustrates the challenging decisions patients can sometimes face at the end of life. It also shows the importance of seeking additional support and guidance before making life-altering decisions.

The woman, whom I will call Margaret, had been living on an inpatient hospice unit for several weeks. She had advanced chronic obstructive pulmonary disease and required around-the-clock ventilation through a breathing mask to avoid shortness of breath. I had the privilege of getting to know Margaret over the course of several weeks as chaplain. Typically, when I would stop by to see her, she was sitting up in a recliner and either doing word-search puzzles, watching television, or conversing with her husband who visited daily.

With the mask on and the machine running, Margaret looked perfectly comfortable and could engage in conversation. She always seemed to appreciate visitors. I would pray with her and bring her Communion

---

24. For a discussion of the Terri Schiavo case in light of Catholic teachings, see Bobby Schindler, "Terri Schiavo, the Brain Injured and Church Teaching," *National Catholic Register*, March 8, 2020, https://www.ncregister.com/blog/terri-schiavo-the-brain-injured-and-church-teaching.

daily, and we would sometimes talk for longer about the Catholic faith, her family, or current events. Our visits were peace filled and joyful.

As chaplain, I was not thoroughly familiar with the details of her case, but I did hear bits and pieces when the interdisciplinary team met. The main reason Margaret needed inpatient hospice as opposed to home hospice was that she did not have enough help at home to consistently manage the breathing machine. It had stopped working several times at home, which was traumatizing for her. Even at inpatient hospice with constant staff monitoring, Margaret continued to struggle with anxiety over the possibility that the machine might fail her again—and that she might die from the lack of air.

From the hospice facility's point of view, Margaret was a delight to care for, but the overall cost of renting and maintaining the ventilator—not to mention the cost of staffing and medications—was higher than Medicare's daily reimbursement rate. In other words, the facility was losing money as they continued caring for her. That is not to say that financial motives directly influenced her plan of care, but the problem of cost was on the radar.

Eventually, the attending who took over Margaret's care started having conversations with her about coming off the breathing machine. Several staff members immediately expressed alarm, because something about it did not seem right. Margaret was doing quite well with the current setup. Her only anxiety, it seemed, was over the possibility of suffocating to death. The fact that she had not initiated these conversations about withdrawing the ventilator mask raised red flags for some of the nurses and myself. Also, no one else was present to observe what was said between the attending and Margaret.

A few days later, I learned that Margaret had agreed to set a date to come off the breathing machine and to be kept comfortable with medications as she took her last breaths. Frankly, I was not quite sure how to handle this situation without crossing a line. I made sure the nursing director was aware and that the ethics committee was consulted. I also brought it up once or twice with Margaret during a visit—gently urging her that she need not feel pressured into doing this. She did not seem to want to talk about it though, as if she had already made up her mind.

Unfortunately, my time as chaplain ended before the date arrived for the removal of Margaret's ventilator mask. I prayed for her regularly and was consoled at least by the idea that Margaret was not at all of a suicidal mindset. She was simply agreeing to a professional recommendation that in many other contexts would be perfectly reasonable. But I could not shake the conviction that, in her case, this was not the right thing to do: Margaret was made to feel that her life was not worth the cost of renting and maintaining the ventilator.

Several days later, I happened to be giving a talk on physician-assisted suicide at a nearby parish—but I decided not to mention anything about my recent experience with Margaret. Afterward, a woman approached me and introduced herself as one of the overnight nurses at the hospice where I had been serving as chaplain. Without any prompting, she told me she was the nurse caring for Margaret the night she died—in other words, Margaret died *overnight*, just hours before she was supposed to come off the ventilator. The nurse assured me that Margaret passed peacefully and with the breathing mask on! I was relieved to hear this and prayed in thanksgiving to God for mercifully sparing this woman in her final hour.

A Twofold Longing

In the above cases, Joe and Margaret had several things in common. They were practicing Catholics who prayed and received the sacraments in their final days. They chose to receive hospice care but also continued to use a breathing machine—an intervention that many patients would find excessively burdensome and, therefore, disproportionate. They encountered a challenging decision point, prompted by their respective attendings, about whether to maintain or withdraw life-sustaining treatment.

A unifying question for Joe and Margaret is this: Should Catholic patients who have advanced illness and are preparing for eternal life with God be more disposed to forgo life-sustaining treatments than Joe and Margaret were, or might there be an important role for some individuals to continue preparing for death as they gradually decline with the aid of life-sustaining treatments? A passage from St. Paul comes to mind: "For to me life is Christ, and death is gain. If I go on living in the flesh, that means fruitful labor for me. And I do not know which I shall choose. I am caught between the two" (Phil. 1:21–23, NABRE).

For some patients at the end of life, it is perfectly clear that life-sustaining interventions are excessively burdensome and inappropriate. The path for them is certain—they do not have long to remain in the flesh before they depart this life and are with Christ. But for others, their path still may be one of fruitful labor in the flesh. Like Paul, their spiritual disposition may be one of equipoise between life with Christ in this world and the gain of eternal life in death. So long as Christ is magnified in their bodies, whether by life or by death, there is cause for rejoicing.

Acknowledgements

The volume editor would like to thank all the
contributors for their chapters.

Special thanks to the staff and editors of the
National Catholic Bioethics Center for
their help preparing this volume.

About the National Catholic Bioethics Center

The National Catholic Bioethics Center (NCBC) is an independent, non-profit, academic research institute dedicated to applying Catholic moral theology and ethical tradition to bioethical questions. Our society faces unprecedented scientific developments that touch upon the mysteries of life and pose serious ethical challenges. The NCBC was established in 1972 to reflect on these issues and to promote and safeguard the dignity of the human person in health care and the life sciences. The NCBC is governed by a board of directors composed of Catholic cardinals and bishops and prominent Catholic pro-life laity. At the heart of the NCBC is its team of expert ethicists, who are assisted by a dedicated support staff, fellows, interns, and members and other benefactors. All of the NCBC's work is done in conformity with the official teachings of the Catholic Church, teachings drawn from a moral tradition that acknowledges the unity of faith and reason and builds on the solid foundation of the natural law.

The NCBC provides consultation on Catholic institutional ethics and witness to many US bishops, the US Conference of Catholic Bishops, Catholic health care systems and hospitals, dicasteries of the Holy See, and international nonprofit health care and social service organizations. NCBC ethicists also respond to individuals' telephone and email questions 24-7, fielding over fifteen hundred consults every year from patients, family members, and health care professionals facing difficult medical decisions. Further, the NCBC offers educational training programs in the Catholic moral tradition and its application to clinical and research situations. Finally, the NCBC is a leading publisher of books and articles on Catholic health care ethics and produces a wide range of electronic resources for professionals and the public.

The NCBC envisions a world in which the integral understanding of the human person underlying Catholic teaching on respect for human life and dignity is better understood and more widely embraced in America and worldwide. For more information, visit the NCBC's website at www.ncbcenter.org.

Printed in the USA
CPSIA information can be obtained
at www.ICGtesting.com
JSHW010849250824
68565JS00007B/32